THE GLP-1 OPTIMIZED HIGH-PROTEIN KETO RESET COOKBOOK

Strategic Eating for Weight Loss & Muscle Retention

Dr. Ben Bigs, PhD

Copyright © 2026

Harbour House Press

harbourhousepublishing.com

TABLE OF CONTENT

TABLE OF CONTENT...3

INTRODUCTION...9

MEDICAL DISCLAIMER...................................... 12

CHAPTER ONE..13

SIMPLE & EASY KETOGENIC COOKING.................. 13

GUIDELINES FOR THE KETOGENIC DIET.................18

KITCHEN EQUIPMENT...................................... 22

THE KETO KITCHEN: WHAT TO EAT, WHAT TO AVOID, AND HOW TO SUCCEED.................................26

FOODS TO AVOID... 31

KETO PANTRY ESSENTIALS................................ 34

FAVORITE KETO PRODUCTS................................36

KETO COOKING MADE SIMPLE............................37

ABOUT THE RECIPES....................................... 38

CHAPTER 2...41

SMOOTHIES & BREAKFASTS...............................41

BULLETPROOF COFFEE.....................................43

BERRY-AVOCADO SMOOTHIE..............................45

ALMOND BUTTER SMOOTHIE............................. 47

BLACKBERRY–CHIA PUDDING............................49

DOUBLE-PORK FRITTATA...................................51

SAUSAGE BREAKFAST STACKS........................... 53

SPICY BREAKFAST SCRAMBLE............................ 55

BACON–JALAPEÑO EGG CUPS............................56

BACON AND EGG CAULIFLOWER HASH..................57

BACON, SPINACH & AVOCADO EGG WRAP..............58

SMOKED SALMON & CREAM CHEESE ROLL-UPS...60

BRUSSELS SPROUTS, BACON & EGGS......................62

BLT BREAKFAST SALAD.. 63

CHEESY EGG & SPINACH NEST.................................. 64

KALE–AVOCADO EGG SKILLET................................. 65

EGG-IN-A-HOLE BREAKFAST BURGER.....................66

PANCAKE "CAKE".. 67

BREAKFAST QUESADILLA..69

CREAM CHEESE MUFFINS.. 72

CHAPTER 3...74

HEARTY SOUPS & SALADS.......................................74

CREAMY TOMATO-BASIL SOUP................................ 76

BROCCOLI-CHEESE SOUP.. 78

CHEESY CAULIFLOWER SOUP....................................80

TACO SOUP... 80

COCONUT AND CAULIFLOWER CURRY SHRIMP
SOUP..81

ROASTED BRUSSELS SPROUTS SALAD WITH
PARMESAN...82

BLT WEDGE SALAD.. 84

MEXICAN EGG SALAD..86

BLUE CHEESE AND BACON KALE SALAD.............89

CHOPPED GREEK SALAD.. 91

MEDITERRANEAN CUCUMBER SALAD....................93

AVOCADO EGG SALAD LETTUCE CUPS.................. 95

AVOCADO CAPRESE SALAD..98

SHRIMP AND AVOCADO SALAD................................100

SALMON CAESAR SALAD... 102

SALMON AND SPINACH COBB SALAD.................. 103

TACO SALAD.. 104

CHEESEBURGER SALAD.. 104

CALIFORNIA STEAK SALAD.....................................105

SKIRT STEAK COBB SALAD..........107

CHAPTER 4............110

SIDE DISHES & SNACKS............110

ROASTED CAULIFLOWER WITH PROSCIUTTO, CAPERS, AND ALMONDS............110

BUTTERY SLOW-COOKER MUSHROOMS............113

BAKED ZUCCHINI GRATIN............115

ROASTED RADISHES WITH BROWN BUTTER SAUCE 117

PARMESAN AND PORK RIND GREEN BEANS.........119

PESTO CAULIFLOWER STEAKS............121

TOMATO, AVOCADO, AND CUCUMBER SALAD.....123

CRUNCHY PORK RIND ZUCCHINI STICKS............125

CHEESE CHIPS AND GUACAMOLE............127

CAULIFLOWER "POTATO" SALAD............129

LOADED CAULIFLOWER MASHED "POTATOES"...131

KETO BREAD............133

DEVILED EGGS............135

CHICKEN-PECAN SALAD CUCUMBER BITES.........138

BUFFALO CHICKEN DIP............140

ROASTED BRUSSELS SPROUTS WITH BACON.......142

SALAMI, PEPPERONCINI, AND CREAM CHEESE PINWHEELS............144

CAULIFLOWER STEAKS WITH BACON AND BLUE CHEESE............146

BACON-WRAPPED JALAPEÑOS............148

CREAMY BROCCOLI-BACON SALAD............150

CHAPTER 5............152

FISH & POULTRY ENTRÉES............152

BAKED LEMON-BUTTER FISH............154

FISH TACO BOWL..155

SCALLOPS WITH CREAMY BACON SAUCE............157

SHRIMP AND AVOCADO LETTUCE CUPS.................158

GARLIC BUTTER SHRIMP.......................................158

PARMESAN-GARLIC SALMON WITH ASPARAGUS159

SEARED SALMON SHIRATAKI RICE BOWLS...........160

PORK RIND SALMON CAKES...................................163

CREAMY DILL SALMON...165

CHICKEN-BASIL ALFREDO WITH SHIRATAKI
NOODLES...167

CHICKEN QUESADILLA...169

GARLIC-PARMESAN CHICKEN WINGS...................170

CHICKEN SKEWERS WITH PEANUT SAUCE...........172

BRAISED CHICKEN THIGHS WITH KALAMATA
OLIVES..174

BUTTERY GARLIC CHICKEN..................................176

CHEESY BACON AND BROCCOLI CHICKEN...........178

PARMESAN BAKED CHICKEN................................179

CRUNCHY CHICKEN MILANESE............................180

BAKED GARLIC AND PAPRIKA CHICKEN LEGS....180

CREAMY SLOW-COOKER CHICKEN.......................181

CHAPTER SIX..182

PORK & BEEF ENTRÉES..182

BLTA CUPS..184

BUTTER AND HERB PORK CHOPS.........................186

PARMESAN PORK CHOPS AND ROASTED
ASPARAGUS...188

SESAME PORK AND GREEN BEANS.......................190

SLOW-COOKER BARBECUE RIBS...........................192

KALUA PORK WITH CABBAGE...............................194

PORK BURGERS WITH SRIRACHA MAYO.............. 196
BLUE CHEESE PORK CHOPS........................197
CARNITAS.. 199
CARNITAS NACHOS...................................200
PEPPERONI LOW-CARB TORTILLA PIZZA.............. 201
BEEF AND BROCCOLI ROAST........................ 202
BEEF AND BELL PEPPER "POTATO SKINS"............. 203
SKIRT STEAK WITH CHIMICHURRI SAUCE........... 206
BARBACOA BEEF ROAST.............................208
STEAK AND EGG BIBIMBAP...........................209
MISSISSIPPI POT ROAST.............................. 212
TACO CHEESE CUPS................................... 214
BACON CHEESEBURGER CASSEROLE....................216
FETA-STUFFED BURGERS.............................. 218
CHAPTER SEVEN.....................................219
DESSERTS & SWEET TREATS..........................219
BLUEBERRY-BLACKBERRY ICE POPS....................220
STRAWBERRY-LIME ICE POPS.........................222
COFFEE ICE POPS..................................... 223
FUDGE ICE POPS.....................................224
ROOT BEER FLOAT................................... 225
ORANGE CREAM FLOAT..............................226
STRAWBERRY SHAKE.................................227
"FROSTY" CHOCOLATE SHAKE.........................228
STRAWBERRY CHEESECAKE MOUSSE...................229
LEMONADE FAT BOMB................................231
BERRY CHEESECAKE FAT BOMB.......................... 232
PEANUT BUTTER FAT BOMB.......................... 233
CHAPTER EIGHT.....................................235
SAUCES & DRESSINGS................................235

DIJON VINAIGRETTE..236
GREEN GODDESS DRESSING...........................237
CAESAR DRESSING...238
AVOCADO-LIME CREMA................................... 239
CHUNKY BLUE CHEESE DRESSING.........................240
SRIRACHA MAYO... 241
AVOCADO MAYO..242
PEANUT SAUCE... 243
GARLIC AIOLI... 244
TZATZIKI... 245
ALFREDO SAUCE.. 247
CONCLUSION.. 249
ABOUT THE AUTHOR..250
REFERENCES...251
RECOMMENDED RESOURCES FOR FURTHER
READING..253

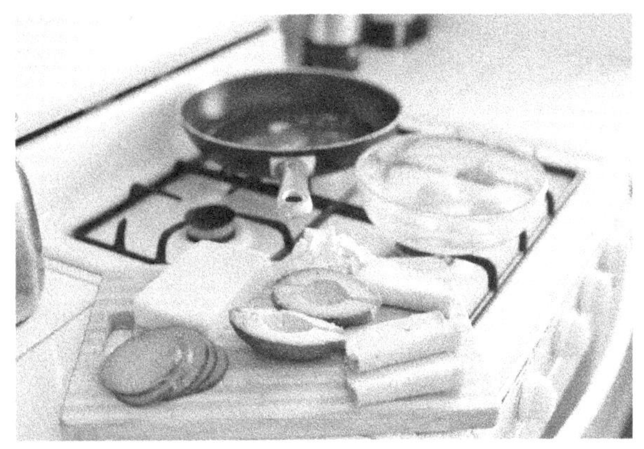

INTRODUCTION

If you're new to keto, you're probably asking the same questions most of us do at the beginning: *What on earth is ketosis? What are macros? And how do I even measure them?* I asked those questions too—and deciding to try the ketogenic lifestyle turned out to be one of the best decisions I've made.

I'm truly glad you're here and that you've chosen to explore this way of eating with me.

The ketogenic diet is a very low-carbohydrate approach that emphasizes healthy fats and moderate protein. While it may feel trendy today, my personal journey with low-carb eating began more than a decade ago, long before "keto" became a buzzword. At the time, I was following the advice of a doctor I was seeing for acupuncture. As a teenager, I had been diagnosed with two autoimmune conditions—psoriatic arthritis and psoriasis—and I was searching for relief from constant pain and inflammation.

His recommendation was simple but life-changing: eliminate sugar.

That was the first time I truly considered the connection between food and how my body feels.

I followed his advice, cut sugar out of my diet, and within weeks I noticed real improvements. The inflammation in my joints eased, and my skin—which had been angry, red, and irritated—began to calm. That experience set me on a path of learning how different foods affect my body and how powerful intentional eating can be.

For many years, I stuck mostly to a low-carbohydrate lifestyle, though like many people, I had seasons where I drifted away from it. A few years ago, my autoimmune symptoms returned, this time more aggressively. Doctors suspected Crohn's disease, but after countless tests and few clear answers, I decided once again to let food be part of my healing process. I focused on high-quality, organic foods and gluten-free carbohydrates. While I saw some improvement, I also felt sluggish—and after six months, I had gained weight thanks to the abundance of tempting gluten-free treats.

That's when I discovered the ketogenic diet.

At first, keto reminded me of the induction phase of the Atkins diet, but something felt different. I loved the focus on real, whole foods, healthy fats, and lower protein. Like many beginners, I felt overwhelmed by the terminology at first—ketosis, macros, net carbs—but I decided to give it an honest try. I'm so glad I did.

Almost immediately, I fell in love with the challenge of creating keto-friendly meals that were quick, simple, and genuinely delicious. As a single mom working full time with a busy teenage daughter, simplicity isn't optional—it's essential. In my experience, you don't need exotic ingredients or a pantry full of specialty oils to eat well on keto.

This book was created for real life.

The recipes inside are designed to help satisfy cravings for the high-carb foods many of us grew up eating. Cravings are completely normal when transitioning to keto—especially if carbohydrates have been a staple in your diet for years. Stick with it. The adjustment is worth it.

My 5-ingredient approach has made keto sustainable for me, and I hope it does the same for you. Most recipes in this book can be prepared in 30 minutes or less, because who honestly has hours to spend in the kitchen? You'll cook with wholesome, affordable ingredients that are easy to find—no specialty grocery store runs required.

Keto doesn't have to be complicated.
It can be simple, satisfying, and enjoyable.

Welcome to Effortless Keto Cooking.

MEDICAL DISCLAIMER

This cookbook is intended for informational and educational purposes only. It is not designed to diagnose, treat, cure, or prevent any medical condition, nor should it be used as a substitute for professional medical advice, diagnosis, or treatment.

Individuals with underlying medical conditions—particularly those affecting glucose regulation, insulin function, metabolic health, or those currently taking GLP-1 receptor agonists or other glucose-lowering medications—should consult their physician, qualified healthcare provider, or registered dietitian before following the ketogenic dietary approaches outlined in this book. Dietary changes may significantly impact blood glucose levels, medication requirements, and overall metabolic stability.

The author and publisher strongly encourage readers to seek personalized medical guidance before making any substantial dietary or lifestyle modifications. Never disregard professional medical advice or delay seeking it because of information contained in this book.

By using this cookbook, you acknowledge that you do so voluntarily and assume full responsibility for your health decisions.

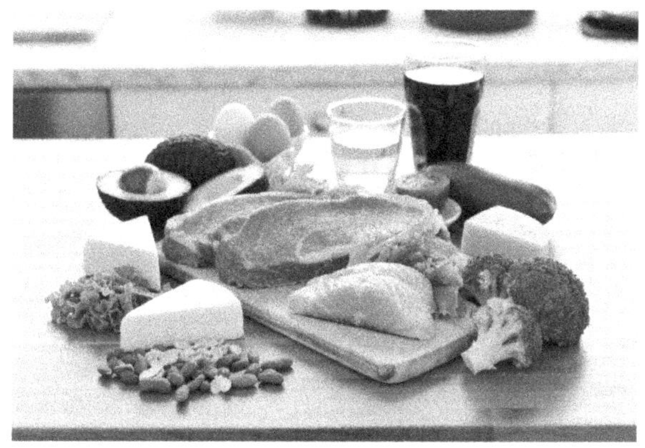

CHAPTER ONE
SIMPLE & EASY KETOGENIC COOKING

One of the things I love most about the ketogenic lifestyle is just how *simple* it can be—both in your own kitchen and when eating out. Keto doesn't require complicated techniques or hard-to-find ingredients. The recipes in this book are built around familiar foods and straightforward methods. I'll show you how to turn everyday ingredients into keto-friendly meals that are satisfying, flavorful, and rich in the healthy fats your body uses for fuel.

The most important step in starting the keto diet is simply this: **start**.
Don't feel intimidated. You don't need to know everything on day one. I'll walk you through the basics so you can feel confident, informed, and ready to succeed.

Why The Keto Diet Works
Beginning a new way of eating can feel overwhelming. I remember the early days of researching keto online—there were charts, formulas, and unfamiliar terms everywhere,

and at times it felt like being back in a science class. But at its core, keto is surprisingly simple.

The ketogenic diet focuses on:

- Healthy fats

- Moderate protein

- Very low carbohydrates

Most of the carbohydrates you do eat come from vegetables. When carbs and sugar are drastically reduced, your body shifts from burning glucose for energy to burning fat. This metabolic state is known as **ketosis**.

Ketosis places your body in an optimal fat-burning mode, which is why keto is so effective for weight loss. But weight loss is only one of many benefits. People often report improved mental clarity, reduced inflammation, steady energy levels, and better overall well-being.

Learning to Listen to Your Body
When you first begin keto, you may notice that you're eating more frequently just to feel full. That's completely normal. As your body becomes accustomed to using fat for fuel—a process called becoming *keto-adapted*—your hunger naturally decreases.

Over time, you may find that you're simply not hungry at traditional mealtimes. I still remind myself of this often. During the workweek, it's easy to eat just because it's "lunchtime." On weekends, without a schedule, I sometimes don't feel hungry until mid-afternoon. Listen to your body. If you're not hungry, you don't need to eat.

That said, hydration is essential. Be sure you're drinking plenty of water and maintaining proper electrolyte balance, especially in the early stages of keto.

Benefits Beyond Weight Loss
Everyone comes to keto for different reasons. For me, reducing inflammation was the priority. Eliminating sugar—one of the most inflammatory substances in the modern diet—has been truly life-changing.

Nutritional ketosis has also been studied for its potential benefits in conditions such as obesity, epilepsy, neurological disorders, and metabolic dysfunction. Becoming a fat burner instead of a sugar burner may even support long-term health and longevity. Research on ketogenic nutrition continues to grow, with new studies emerging regularly.

Common Keto Questions, Made Simple
What is ketosis?
Ketosis occurs when carbohydrate intake is kept very low, prompting the liver to convert fat into fatty acids and ketone bodies. These ketones become the body's primary energy source, including for the brain. Most people enter ketosis within the first week of starting keto, though full keto-adaptation typically takes several weeks.

What are macros, and why do they matter?
Macros—short for macronutrients—are the main components of food that provide calories: fat, protein, and carbohydrates.

The standard American diet averages:

- 50% carbohydrates

- 15% protein

- 35% fat

A typical ketogenic macro ratio looks more like:

- 5% carbohydrates

- 20–25% protein

- 70–75% fat

To determine your personal macros, you can use an online keto macro calculator. These tools consider your height, weight, activity level, and goals to provide daily targets for calories, fat, protein, and carbohydrates. For weight loss, many people aim to stay under **20 net carbs per day**, which is also my personal target.

Tracking apps like *Carb Manager* can make this process easy and help you monitor net carbs.

What are net carbs?
Net carbs are calculated by subtracting fiber from total carbohydrates, since fiber isn't digested by the body. For example, if a food contains 3 grams of total carbs and 1 gram of fiber, the net carb count is 2 grams.

Some people track total carbs, others track net carbs—both approaches can work. Choose the method that feels most sustainable for you.

Is eating that much fat really healthy?
Eating a high-fat diet may feel counterintuitive at first, especially if you're used to low-fat messaging. The key is focusing on **high-quality fats**. Grass-fed butter and meats, ghee, full-fat dairy, avocados, nuts, olive oil, and fatty fish like salmon are all excellent choices. Low-quality industrial oils, such as vegetable and canola oils, should be avoided.

Quality fats promote satiety, which is why keto naturally reduces hunger.

What is intermittent fasting?
Intermittent fasting (IF) pairs well with a ketogenic lifestyle. Many people follow a 16:8 approach—fasting for

16 hours and eating within an 8-hour window. For example, eating between noon and 8 p.m.

During fasting periods, non-caloric beverages like water are encouraged. Some people also include fat-based drinks such as Bulletproof Coffee, which can help curb appetite while remaining keto-friendly.

What does keto-adapted mean?
While ketosis can begin within days, becoming keto-adapted takes longer. Once adapted, your body efficiently uses fat as its primary fuel source instead of glucose. This transition typically occurs after several weeks of consistently following ketogenic macros.

GUIDELINES FOR THE KETOGENIC DIET

Transitioning your body from burning glucose to burning fat is a significant metabolic shift. With any major change comes a period of adjustment, so it's important to support your body during this transition. When starting a ketogenic diet, focus on nutrient-dense foods, adequate hydration, balanced electrolytes, and plenty of rest. This is a healing phase, and your body needs time to adapt.

Electrolytes play a vital role in nearly every bodily function. They help regulate muscle contractions, nerve signals, heart rhythm, and cellular balance. When electrolytes are depleted or out of balance, you may feel fatigued, weak, or generally "off."

Managing Electrolytes and the "Keto Flu"

As your body flushes out stored carbohydrates and sugar, it also releases water and electrolytes. This process—often referred to as the *keto flu*—is temporary, but it can cause symptoms such as headaches, lightheadedness, muscle cramps, nausea, and fatigue.

The good news is that these symptoms can usually be minimized by intentionally managing your electrolytes.

Helpful strategies include:

- Drink plenty of water with added electrolytes.

- Increase your salt intake using high-quality salt, such as pink Himalayan salt.

- Sip bone broth or vegetable broth as needed.

- Eat potassium-rich, low-carb foods like avocados and leafy greens.

- Include magnesium-rich foods such as nuts, spinach, artichokes, and fish.

- Prioritize rest—your body is adjusting and healing.

Staying consistent through this phase is key. The discomfort is temporary, but the benefits are long-lasting.

Hydration Is Non-Negotiable
Proper hydration is essential throughout your ketogenic journey. In the early stages of keto, your body sheds a significant amount of water because carbohydrates naturally cause water retention. As those carbs are removed, your body releases that excess water—making replenishment critical.

A simple guideline is to drink **at least half your body weight in ounces of water each day**. For example, if you weigh 200 pounds, aim for a minimum of 100 ounces of water daily. Adjust upward based on activity level, climate, and personal needs.

Don't Fear Salt
On a standard high-carbohydrate diet, many processed foods already contain large amounts of sodium. On keto, those foods are eliminated, so you'll need to be more intentional about adding salt back into your meals.

Season your food generously with high-quality salt, and if needed, supplement with broth. Pink Himalayan salt is an excellent option because it contains trace minerals such as potassium, magnesium, and iron—minerals that are especially important on a ketogenic diet.

Easy Ways to Increase Healthy Fats
Reaching 70–75 percent of your daily calories from fat may sound intimidating at first, but it doesn't have to be

complicated. The simplest approach is to consistently add healthy fats to the foods you're already eating.

Butter, olive oil, avocado oil, coconut oil, and full-fat dairy can easily be incorporated into meals. A little added fat goes a long way in keeping you full, satisfied, and energized.

Eating Keto When Dining Out
One of the most practical advantages of keto is how adaptable it is when eating out. With a little planning, you can find keto-friendly options at almost any restaurant.

Whenever possible, review the menu online ahead of time. Look for meals centered around meat, fish, eggs, and vegetables. Be cautious with sauces, dressings, and marinades, as they often contain hidden sugars and starches.

When in doubt, ask your server about ingredients or request sauces on the side. Restaurants are accustomed to dietary preferences, so don't hesitate to customize your order.

Ketogenic or Paleo?
Keto and Paleo are often mentioned together, but they are **not the same** eating plan.

A **typical Paleo diet** focuses on whole, unprocessed foods similar to what early humans might have eaten—meat, fish, vegetables, fruits, nuts, and seeds. While Paleo avoids processed foods, it is not as low in carbohydrates or as high in fat as keto. Foods like sweet potatoes and carrots are allowed, and Paleo macros often average around:

- 20% carbohydrates

- 15% protein

- 65% fat

The **ketogenic diet**, on the other hand, requires strict carbohydrate restriction to maintain ketosis. High-carb vegetables and starches are avoided because they raise blood glucose and prevent fat-burning. Keto macros typically fall around:

- 5% carbohydrates

- 20% protein

- 75% fat

Remaining in ketosis is what defines keto—without it, the diet becomes simply low-carb.

What About Dairy?
Dairy is another key difference between the two approaches. On keto, full-fat dairy can be a valuable and convenient source of healthy fats, though it is not mandatory. Traditional Paleo diets avoid dairy altogether, although modern Paleo variations may allow limited forms.

It *is* possible to follow a ketogenic diet while incorporating Paleo principles—especially the emphasis on high-quality, minimally processed foods. When possible, choose the best ingredients you can afford. Simple swaps, such as using ghee instead of butter or coconut milk instead of heavy cream, can help align keto meals with Paleo preferences.

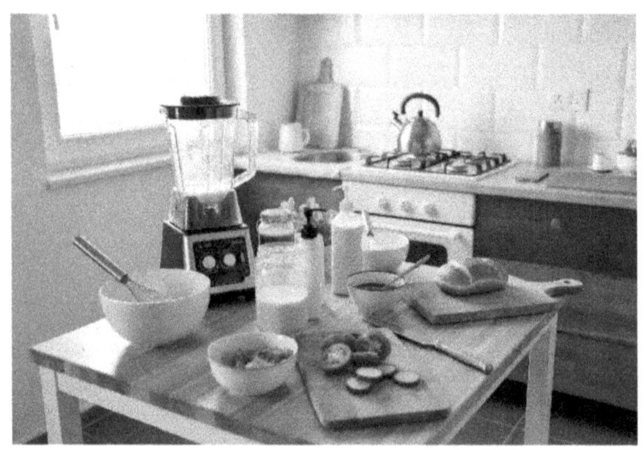

KITCHEN EQUIPMENT

You don't need a kitchen full of fancy gadgets to make the recipes in this book. However, having a few essential tools on hand will make your cooking easier, faster, and more enjoyable. Here are the key items I recommend for everyday keto cooking:

Must-Have Tools

- **Measuring cups and spoons:** Accurate measurements are important—especially for baking recipes and if you're watching portion sizes for weight loss. Eyeballing ingredients won't always give the best results.

- **Basic utensils:** A spatula, slotted spoon, large spoon, whisk, tongs, and rubber scraper. You only need one of each, and these six tools cover most of your cooking needs.

- **Cutting boards:** Ideally, have two—one for vegetables and another for meat—to keep things sanitary and organized.

- **Knives:** Invest in one or two good-quality chef's knives. A 6-inch chef's knife and a paring knife are a great starting point. You don't need expensive knives, but sharp, reliable ones will make your prep work much easier.

- **Cheese grater/zester:** Grating your own cheese is often cheaper and fresher than buying pre-shredded. Some graters even come with built-in containers for convenience. A citrus zester can also be handy for zesting lemons, limes, and other ingredients.

- **Baking sheet:** A large baking sheet is perfect for roasting vegetables, cooking one-pan meals, or baking.

- **9-by-13-inch baking pan:** A deeper pan works well for roasting meats, vegetables, and making egg frittatas. I love using an easy-to-clean enameled cast-iron pan, like Le Creuset.

- **9-by-5-inch loaf pan:** This is the standard size I use for baking Keto Bread.

- **Muffin tin:** Many recipes call for muffins or mini bites. A standard muffin tin works fine, but a jumbo size can be handy for larger portions, like BLTA Cups.

- **8-inch glass baking dish:** This smaller, deep glass pan is perfect for desserts or cooking smaller batches.

- **10- or 12-inch skillet:** I prefer a nonstick skillet for ease of cooking and cleanup, especially for staples like eggs. While professional chefs might prefer stainless steel for searing, a nonstick pan works beautifully for most keto meals. Whichever you choose, make sure it has a lid.

- **Saucepans:** Having a small (around 2-quart) and a larger (about 4.5-quart) saucepan covers most of your cooking needs.

- **Slow cooker:** A slow cooker is a lifesaver for easy one-pot meals, especially during cooler months. I use a simple 6-quart model without fancy features, and it works like a charm.

- **Colander:** Useful for washing fruits and vegetables. A medium-size colander is usually sufficient unless you're cooking for a crowd.

- **Mixing bowls:** A set of nesting mixing bowls is invaluable. I have mine for over a decade and use them daily.

- **Ice pop molds:** Fun and easy for making keto-friendly ice pops in any shape you like.

- **Parchment paper:** I use parchment paper for everything—from lining pans for egg frittatas to roasting vegetables and making cheese chips. Pre-cut squares save time, and be sure to check the temperature rating (up to 425°F is typical).

- **Blender or food processor:**

  - A **blender** is great for smoothies, soups, coffee drinks, and sauces.

  - A **food processor** is incredibly versatile—I use mine all the time for chopping, mixing, and pureeing. A small model like the Cuisinart Mini-Prep works perfectly for smaller households.

Nice-to-Have Tools

- **Mixer:** Whether it's an electric hand mixer or a countertop stand mixer, this tool is especially helpful for desserts. If you don't have one, a whisk can also do the job—and double as a great arm workout!

- **Kitchen scale:** Not essential, but many keto followers find a scale useful for accurately measuring portions, particularly proteins.

- **Immersion blender:** Perfect for quickly blending soups and sauces right in the pot or bowl without transferring to a blender.

- **Rolling pin:** Handy for rolling out dough or shaping dishes like pinwheels. No rolling pin? A clean wine bottle works just as well!

- **Basting brush:** Great for applying oil evenly. If you don't have one, a leafy green or paper towel can do the trick.

- **Cooling rack:** Useful for letting baked goods cool evenly. If you don't have one, trivets or pot holders work just fine.

THE KETO KITCHEN: WHAT TO EAT, WHAT TO AVOID, AND HOW TO SUCCEED

Foods to Enjoy
High-Fat / Low-Carb Choices (Based on Net Carbs)

A successful ketogenic lifestyle begins with choosing foods that are naturally low in carbohydrates and rich in healthy fats. The following foods form the backbone of simple, satisfying keto meals.

Meats & Seafood
These protein sources are naturally low in carbs and pair beautifully with healthy fats:

- Beef (ground beef, steak, roasts)

- Chicken

- Crab

- Crawfish

- Duck

- Fish (fresh or wild-caught when possible)

- Goose

- Lamb

- Lobster

- Mussels

- Octopus

- Pork (pork chops, bacon, ribs)

- Quail

- Sausage (without fillers or added sugars)

- Scallops

- Shrimp

- Veal

- Venison

Dairy
Choose full-fat, minimally processed options whenever possible:

- Blue cheese dressing

- Burrata cheese

- Cottage cheese (full-fat)

- Cream cheese

- Eggs

- Greek yogurt (full-fat, unsweetened)

- Grilling cheese

- Halloumi cheese

- Heavy (whipping) cream

- Homemade whipped cream

- Kefalotyri cheese

- Mozzarella cheese

- Provolone cheese

- Queso blanco

- Ranch dressing

- Ricotta cheese

- Unsweetened almond milk

- Unsweetened coconut milk

Nuts & Seeds

Enjoy these in moderation, as carbs can add up quickly:

- Almonds

- Brazil nuts

- Chia seeds

- Flaxseeds

- Hazelnuts

- Macadamia nuts

- Peanuts (moderation is key)

- Pecans

- Pine nuts

- Pumpkin seeds

- Sacha inchi seeds

- Sesame seeds

- Walnuts

Fruits & Vegetables

Low-carb vegetables and select fruits add fiber, nutrients, and color to your plate:

- Alfalfa sprouts

- Asparagus

- Avocados

- Bell peppers

- Blackberries

- Blueberries

- Broccoli

- Cabbage

- Carrots (in moderation)

- Cauliflower

- Celery

- Chicory

- Coconut

- Cranberries

- Cucumbers

- Garlic (in moderation)

- Green beans

- Fresh herbs

- Jicama

- Lemons

- Limes
- Mushrooms
- Okra
- Olives
- Onions (in moderation)
- Pickles
- Pumpkin
- Radishes
- Raspberries
- Salad greens
- Scallions
- Spaghetti squash (in moderation)
- Strawberries
- Tomatoes (in moderation)
- Zucchini

FOODS TO AVOID

Low-Fat / High-Carb Foods (Based on Net Carbs)

These foods can quickly push you out of ketosis and make progress difficult. Limiting or eliminating them will greatly support your success.

Meats & Meat Alternatives
- Deli meats (some varieties contain added sugars and fillers)

- Hot dogs (with fillers)

- Sausage (with fillers)

- Seitan

- Tofu

Dairy
- Sweetened almond milk

- Sweetened coconut milk

- Milk

- Soy milk

- Regular yogurt

Nuts & Seeds
- Cashews

- Chestnuts

- Pistachios

Fruits & Vegetables

- Apples

- Apricots

- Artichokes

- Bananas

- Beans (all varieties)

- Boysenberries

- Burdock root

- Butternut squash

- Cantaloupe

- Cherries

- Chickpeas

- Corn

- Currants

- Dates

- Edamame

- Eggplant

- Elderberries

- Gooseberries

- Grapes

- Honeydew melon

- Huckleberries

- Kiwi

- Leeks

- Mangoes

- Oranges

- Parsnips

- Peaches

- Peas

- Pineapple

- Plantains

- Plums

- Potatoes

- Prunes

- Raisins

- Sweet potatoes

- Taro root

- Turnips

- Water chestnuts

- Winter squash

- Yams

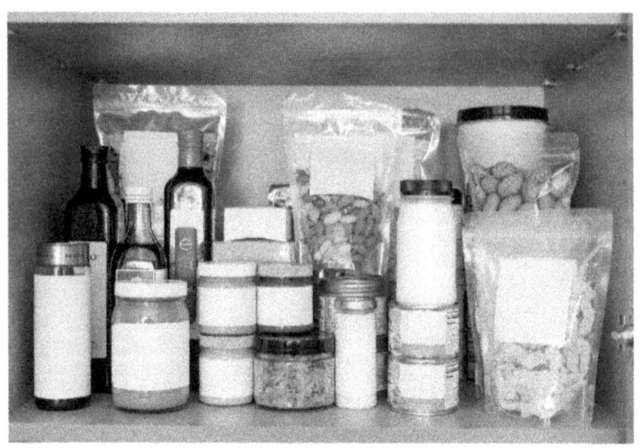

KETO PANTRY ESSENTIALS

Cooking keto does not require exotic or expensive ingredients. Success comes from simplicity and preparation. Each recipe in this book uses only **five main ingredients**, but the following staples do not count toward that total.

Keto Cooking Staples
Keep these five essentials stocked at all times:

1. Pink Himalayan salt

2. Freshly ground black pepper

3. Ghee (clarified butter; grass-fed when possible)

4. Olive oil

5. Grass-fed butter

Keto Perishables
These ingredients are worth keeping on hand for quick meals and snacks. When possible, choose organic or all-natural options.

1. Eggs (pasture-raised, if available)

2. Avocados

3. Bacon (uncured)

4. Cream cheese (full-fat or dairy-free alternative)

5. Sour cream (full-fat or dairy-free alternative)

6. Heavy whipping cream or full-fat canned coconut milk

7. Garlic (fresh or pre-minced)

8. Cauliflower

9. Meat (grass-fed when possible)

10. Greens (spinach, kale, or arugula)

FAVORITE KETO PRODUCTS

Over time, I have found certain products that consistently deliver quality, flavor, and convenience. Some are staples, while others are treats or specialty items. You'll find sourcing details and discounts in the Resources section.

- **Vital Farms Pasture-Raised Eggs**
  Rich yolks, superior taste, and responsibly sourced.

- **Kerrygold Grass-Fed Butter**
  Higher fat content and unmatched flavor.

- **Bulletproof Brain Octane Oil**
  A simple way to boost healthy fat intake without flavor or odor.

- **Bulletproof Ghee**
  High smoke point and dairy-free, perfect for keto cooking.

- **Primal Palate Spice Mixes**
  High-quality seasonings that elevate simple meals.

- **Perfect Keto MCT Oil Powder**
  Mess-free fats with a creamy texture for drinks and baking.

- **Perfect Keto Collagen Protein Powder**
  Supports joints, skin, hair, and nails while remaining keto-friendly.

- **Fat Snax Cookies & Keto Kookies**
  Convenient low-carb treats for occasional indulgence.

- **Trader Joe's Rosemary Marcona Almonds**
  Rich, buttery, and incredibly satisfying.

- **Miracle Noodles & Miracle Rice**
  Zero-net-carb alternatives for classic comfort
  dishes.

- **Primal Kitchen Sauces & Dressings**
  Clean ingredients made with avocado oil and no
  added sugars.

KETO COOKING MADE SIMPLE

The ketogenic diet may seem overwhelming at first, but at its core, it is about simplifying the way you eat. Success comes from choosing real foods, limiting ingredients, and planning ahead.

Each recipe in this book reflects that philosophy. By shopping intentionally and cooking with purpose, you set yourself up for long-term success.

- Use the highest-quality ingredients you can afford.

- Remove non-keto foods from your home.

- Keep meals simple and ingredient lists short.

- Track your food intake to stay mindful of your macros.

- Plan meals and prep ingredients ahead of time.

- Cook in bulk to save time and money.

- Experiment with flavors and seasonings.

- Don't fear salt—your body needs it on keto.

Most importantly, **commit**. It can take several weeks for your body to fully adapt to ketosis. Be patient, consistent, and kind to yourself. Keto is not a quick fix—it is a sustainable way of eating designed to support healing, energy, and long-term health.

ABOUT THE RECIPES

In this book, you will find **130 easy, five-ingredient ketogenic recipes** designed to make everyday cooking simple and enjoyable. These recipes cover every meal of the day, from quick breakfasts to satisfying dinners and treats.

More than half of the recipes can be prepared in **30 minutes or less**, and whenever possible, I've kept the number of pots and pans to a minimum—because great food should not come with a sink full of dishes.

Recipe Labels
To help you quickly find what works best for your schedule and preferences, each recipe includes clear, helpful labels:

- **ONE POT** – Made using a single pot or bowl

- **ONE PAN** – Prepared in one skillet, baking dish, or cooking vessel

- **30-MINUTE** – Ready in 30 minutes or less, including prep and cooking

- **NO COOK** – Requires no cooking at all

- **VEGETARIAN** – Contains no meat

Ingredients & Nutrition
Every recipe uses **just five main ingredients**, along with any combination of the following pantry staples, which do not count toward the ingredient total:

- Pink Himalayan salt

- Freshly ground black pepper

- Grass-fed ghee

- Olive oil

- Grass-fed butter

At the end of each recipe, you'll find **nutritional information and macro breakdowns**, making it easy to track fat, protein, carbohydrates, and calories while staying on plan.

Helpful Tips in Every Recipe
Each recipe also includes at least one helpful tip to make cooking even easier:

- **Substitution Tip** – Suggestions for swapping ingredients based on preference or availability

- **Ingredient Tip** – Simple or alternative ways to prepare ingredients

- **Variations** – Easy ideas for changing flavors or ingredients while keeping the recipe keto-friendly

Serving Size

Most recipes are designed to serve **two people**. I originally developed these meals for myself and my daughter, and I've since learned that two-person portions are a favorite among readers. If you're cooking for more people, simply multiply the ingredients to suit your needs.

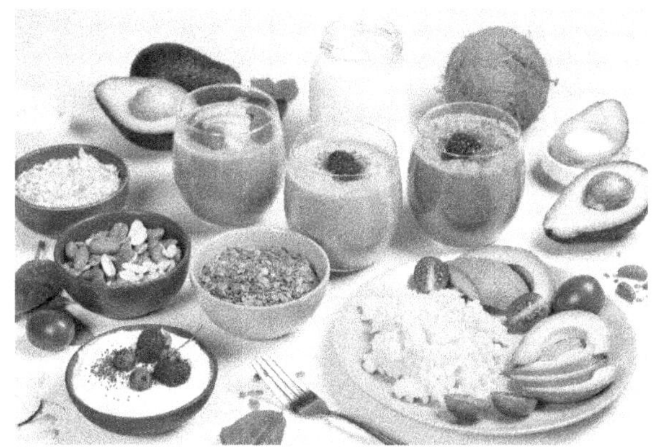

CHAPTER 2
SMOOTHIES & BREAKFASTS

The ketogenic diet and breakfast go hand in hand. With just one ingredient—**eggs**—there are countless ways to get creative, satisfying, and delicious. The recipes in this chapter are some of my personal favorites, many of which I regularly make for my daughter and myself.

During busy work and school mornings, I usually keep breakfast simple with **Bulletproof Coffee** or an **Americano with heavy whipping cream**. On weekends, however, I enjoy taking a little more time to prepare hearty keto breakfasts we can truly savor.

This chapter will show you how to transform classic morning favorites—like carb-heavy smoothies and pancakes—into **easy, low-carb, keto-friendly alternatives** that still feel indulgent and comforting.

Recipes in This Chapter
- Bulletproof Coffee

- Berry-Avocado Smoothie

- Almond Butter Smoothie

- Blackberry-Chia Pudding

- Double-Pork Frittata

- Sausage Breakfast Stacks

- Spicy Breakfast Scramble

- Bacon–Jalapeño Egg Cups

- Bacon and Egg Cauliflower Hash

- Bacon, Spinach, and Avocado Egg Wrap

- Smoked Salmon and Cream Cheese Roll-Ups

- Brussels Sprouts, Bacon, and Eggs

- BLT Breakfast Salad

- Cheesy Egg and Spinach Nest

- Kale-Avocado Egg Skillet

- Egg-in-a-Hole Breakfast Burger

- Cream Cheese and Coconut Flour Pancakes or Waffles

- Pancake "Cake"

- Breakfast Quesadilla

- Cream Cheese Muffins

BULLETPROOF COFFEE

Bulletproof Coffee is a staple beverage in many ketogenic lifestyles—and for good reason. I love how energized and focused I feel after drinking it; honestly, it makes me feel like **Wonder Woman**. One of the biggest benefits is that the high fat content helps me extend my **intermittent fast**, keeping me satisfied until lunchtime.

If you're not using Bulletproof Coffee for fasting, you can easily add protein or collagen to make it a more filling breakfast option.

30-MINUTE | ONE PAN | NO COOK
SERVES: 1
PREP TIME: 5 minutes

Ingredients
- 1½ cups hot coffee

- 2 tablespoons MCT oil powder *or* Bulletproof Brain Octane Oil

- 2 tablespoons butter or ghee

Instructions
1. Pour the hot coffee into a blender.

2. Add the oil powder and butter, then blend until frothy and fully combined.

3. Pour into a large mug and enjoy immediately.

Variations
If you're not intermittent fasting and want to add protein, try one of the following:

- **Raw egg:** Replace the MCT oil powder with 1 raw egg for added protein and creaminess. The hot coffee gently cooks the egg, leaving no eggy taste.

- **Protein or collagen powder:** Add one or two scoops of protein powder. Perfect Keto Collagen is a favorite, especially the chocolate flavor.

- **Spiced:** Add 1 teaspoon cinnamon and a keto-friendly sweetener for a warm, spiced version.

Ingredient Tip:
If you're new to keto, start slowly with Brain Octane Oil. It's very potent—gradually work your way up to 2 tablespoons over a few weeks.

Per Serving:
Calories: 463 | Fat: 51g | Carbs: 0g | Net Carbs: 0g | Fiber: 0g | Protein: 1g

BERRY-AVOCADO SMOOTHIE

This smoothie is one of my all-time favorites. It's rich, creamy, and packed with healthy fats, fiber, potassium, and magnesium. Add liquid stevia if you prefer a sweeter smoothie.

30-MINUTE | ONE PAN | NO COOK | VEGETARIAN
SERVES: 2
PREP TIME: 5 minutes

Ingredients
- 1 cup unsweetened full-fat coconut milk

- 1 scoop Perfect Keto Exogenous Ketone Powder (Peaches & Cream)

- ½ avocado

- 1 cup fresh spinach

- ½ cup berries (fresh or frozen, no sugar added)

- ½ cup ice cubes

- ¼ teaspoon liquid stevia (optional)

Instructions
1. Add all ingredients to a blender.

2. Blend until smooth, creamy, and frothy.

3. Pour into tall glasses and enjoy.

Ingredient Tip:
Avocado adds healthy fats and nutrients while giving the smoothie a luxuriously creamy texture.

Per Batch:
Calories: 709 | Fat: 68g | Carbs: 27g | Net Carbs: 14g |
Fiber: 12g | Protein: 8g

Per Serving:
Calories: 355 | Fat: 40g | Carbs: 16g | Net Carbs: 8g | Fiber:
6g | Protein: 4g

ALMOND BUTTER SMOOTHIE

When I make this smoothie, my daughter feels like she's drinking a milkshake—yet it's incredibly nourishing. I love knowing she's enjoying something delicious that also fuels her body and mind for hours. Add liquid stevia if you prefer extra sweetness.

30-MINUTE | ONE PAN | NO COOK | VEGETARIAN
SERVES: 2
PREP TIME: 5 minutes

Ingredients
- 1 cup unsweetened full-fat coconut milk
- 1 scoop Perfect Keto Exogenous Ketone Powder (Chocolate Sea Salt)
- ½ avocado
- 2 tablespoons almond butter
- ½ cup berries (fresh or frozen, no sugar added)
- ½ cup ice cubes
- ¼ teaspoon liquid stevia (optional)

Instructions
1. Combine all ingredients in a blender.
2. Blend until smooth and creamy.
3. Serve immediately in tall glasses.

Ingredient Tip:
For added nutrition, try:

- 1 teaspoon turmeric powder for anti-inflammatory benefits, or

- 1 tablespoon chia seeds soaked in coconut milk for at least 20 minutes to boost fiber, calcium, iron, and omega-3s.

Per Batch:
Calories: 892 | Fat: 85g | Carbs: 31g | Net Carbs: 17g | Fiber: 14g | Protein: 14g

Per Serving:
Calories: 446 | Fat: 43g | Carbs: 16g | Net Carbs: 9g | Fiber: 7g | Protein: 7g

BLACKBERRY–CHIA PUDDING

This recipe came together on a day when I spotted a lone can of coconut milk in my pantry and wanted to turn it into something new. After asking my Instagram community for ideas, chia pudding was the winning suggestion. I paired it with blackberries—a fantastic low-carb fruit that adds both vibrant flavor and texture.

While this pudding easily doubles as a dessert, I often enjoy it for breakfast. Chia seeds are nutritional powerhouses, packed with fiber, iron, calcium, and omega-3 fatty acids. Once soaked overnight, they absorb the coconut milk, soften, and naturally thicken the pudding. The combination of healthy fats and fiber slows digestion and keeps you feeling full for hours.

ONE PAN • NO COOK • VEGETARIAN
Serves: 2
Prep Time: 10 minutes, plus overnight to set

Ingredients

- 1 cup unsweetened full-fat coconut milk
- 1 teaspoon liquid stevia
- 1 teaspoon vanilla extract
- ½ cup blackberries (fresh or frozen, no sugar added)
- ¼ cup chia seeds

Instructions

1. In a food processor or blender, blend the coconut milk, stevia, and vanilla until slightly thickened.

2. Add the blackberries and blend until fully combined and vibrantly purple.
3. Fold in the chia seeds.
4. Divide the mixture between two small lidded containers and refrigerate overnight or up to 3 days before serving.

Cooking Tip
Blending is essential. Whisking by hand will not properly thicken the mixture.

Nutrition (Per Serving)
Calories: 437 • Fat: 38g • Net Carbs: 8g • Fiber: 15g • Protein: 8g

DOUBLE-PORK FRITTATA

Frittatas are one of my favorite make-ahead keto breakfasts. I used to rely on cheese for richness until one day I ran out and substituted heavy cream instead. The result was so fluffy and satisfying that I never looked back.

This version features two types of pork—pancetta and prosciutto—for deep, savory flavor. I recommend using high-quality pork lard or reserved bacon fat, but butter works beautifully as well.

30-MINUTE
Serves: 4
Prep: 5 minutes • Cook: 25 minutes

Ingredients

- 1 tablespoon butter or pork lard
- 8 large eggs
- 1 cup heavy whipping cream
- Pink Himalayan salt
- Freshly ground black pepper
- 4 oz pancetta, chopped
- 2 oz prosciutto, thinly sliced
- 1 tablespoon fresh dill, chopped

Instructions

1. Preheat the oven to 375°F (190°C). Grease a 9×13-inch baking dish.
2. In a large bowl, whisk the eggs and cream until smooth. Season with salt and pepper.

3. Pour into the prepared dish and evenly scatter the pancetta throughout.
4. Tear the prosciutto into pieces and place on top. Sprinkle with dill.
5. Bake for about 25 minutes, until the edges are golden and the center is just set.
6. Let cool for 5 minutes before slicing and serving.

Variation Ideas

- Sausage and fresh spinach
- Bacon, mushrooms, and spinach
- Ham, green peppers, and scallions

Cooking Tip

For individual servings, bake in a greased muffin tin to create egg bites.

SAUSAGE BREAKFAST STACKS

Keto breakfasts shine when simple ingredients come together beautifully. Juicy sausage patties layered with mashed avocado and topped with a sunny-side-up egg make for a hearty, satisfying start to the day.

30-MINUTE
Serves: 2
Prep: 10 minutes • Cook: 15 minutes

Ingredients

- 8 oz ground pork
- ½ teaspoon garlic powder
- ½ teaspoon onion powder
- 2 tablespoons ghee, divided
- 2 large eggs
- 1 avocado
- Pink Himalayan salt
- Freshly ground black pepper

Instructions

1. Preheat the oven to 375°F (190°C).
2. Combine the pork with garlic and onion powders. Form into two patties.
3. Heat 1 tablespoon ghee in a skillet and brown patties for 2 minutes per side.
4. Transfer to a baking sheet and bake 8–10 minutes, until cooked through.
5. In the same skillet, melt remaining ghee and fry the eggs sunny-side-up.
6. Mash the avocado and season lightly.

7. Assemble by stacking sausage, avocado, and egg. Serve immediately.

Substitution Tip
Use sugar-free frozen sausage patties for a faster option.

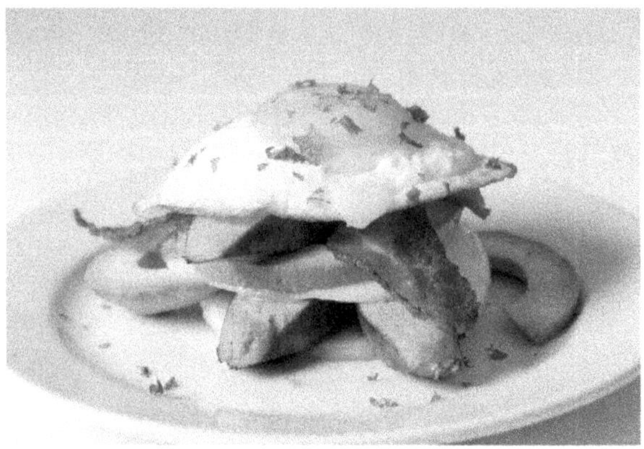

SPICY BREAKFAST SCRAMBLE

This bold, Mexican-inspired scramble combines spicy chorizo with creamy eggs and melted cheese. It's endlessly adaptable and keeps you full well into the day.

30-MINUTE
Serves: 2
Prep: 5 minutes • Cook: 10 minutes

Ingredients

- 2 tablespoons ghee
- 6 oz Mexican chorizo (or spicy sausage)
- 6 large eggs
- 2 tablespoons heavy cream
- Pink Himalayan salt
- Freshly ground black pepper
- ½ cup shredded pepper Jack cheese, divided
- ½ cup chopped scallions

Instructions

1. Melt ghee in a skillet and brown the sausage until fully cooked.
2. Whisk eggs with cream, salt, and pepper.
3. Push sausage to one side and pour eggs into the skillet.
4. When nearly set, stir in half the cheese.
5. Combine eggs and sausage, top with remaining cheese and scallions, and serve.

BACON–JALAPEÑO EGG CUPS

These portable egg cups are perfect for breakfast, snacks, or meal prep. Crispy bacon forms the shell, while cream cheese and jalapeño add richness and heat.

30-MINUTE
Makes: 6 egg cups

Ingredients

- 6 bacon slices
- 1 tablespoon butter
- 2 jalapeños
- 4 large eggs
- 2 oz cream cheese, softened
- Pink Himalayan salt
- Black pepper
- ¼ cup shredded Mexican-blend cheese

Instructions

1. Preheat oven to 375°F (190°C).
2. Partially cook bacon, then line greased muffin cups.
3. Beat eggs, cream cheese, minced jalapeño, salt, and pepper.
4. Fill cups two-thirds full, top with cheese and jalapeño rings.
5. Bake 20 minutes. Cool slightly before serving.

BACON AND EGG CAULIFLOWER HASH

Cauliflower replaces potatoes in this one-skillet breakfast, delivering all the comfort without the carbs. It's quick, filling, and full of flavor.

30-MINUTE • ONE PAN
Serves: 2

Instructions

1. Cook bacon until crisp. Chop and set aside.
2. Sauté cauliflower, onion, and garlic in bacon fat until lightly browned.
3. Create wells and crack eggs into the pan.
4. Season, cook until eggs set, top with bacon, and serve.

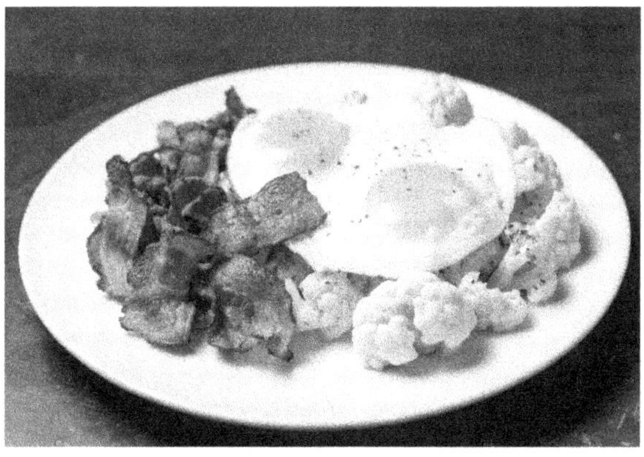

BACON, SPINACH & AVOCADO EGG WRAP

One morning, while planning to make a simple omelet, the idea of turning the eggs into a wrap came to mind. Cooked like a thin, flat omelet, the egg acts as a crêpe or tortilla, perfectly enclosing a variety of fillings. Egg wraps are incredibly versatile, and for this version, I filled them with crispy bacon, fresh spinach, and creamy avocado.

30-MINUTE
Serves: 2
Prep: 10 minutes
Cook: 10 minutes

Ingredients

- 6 bacon slices
- 2 large eggs
- 2 tablespoons heavy whipping cream
- Pink salt
- Freshly ground black pepper
- 1 tablespoon butter (if needed)
- 1 cup fresh spinach (or greens of choice)
- ½ avocado, sliced

Instructions

1. Heat a medium skillet over medium-high heat and cook the bacon until crispy, about 8 minutes. Transfer to a paper towel–lined plate.
2. In a medium bowl, whisk together the eggs and cream. Season with pink salt and black pepper.

3. Pour half of the egg mixture into the skillet with the bacon grease.
4. Cook for about 1 minute, until set, then carefully flip and cook the other side for another minute.
5. Transfer to a paper towel–lined plate to absorb excess grease.
6. Repeat with the remaining egg mixture, adding butter if the pan becomes dry.
7. Place one egg wrap on each warm plate. Top evenly with spinach, bacon, and avocado.
8. Season lightly, roll into wraps, and serve hot.

Variations

- Add chopped romaine lettuce for a fresh crunch alongside bacon and tomato.
- For extra heat, mix diced jalapeños or hot sauce into the egg batter and fill with sausage and shredded cheese.

Substitution Tip
To make these wraps dairy-free, omit the cream and use one additional egg.

SMOKED SALMON & CREAM CHEESE ROLL-UPS

Though typically served as appetizers, these salmon roll-ups make a surprisingly satisfying breakfast. Inspired by classic bagels and lox, they deliver all the familiar flavors—without the carbohydrates.

30-MINUTE • ONE POT • NO COOK
Serves: 2
Prep: 25 minutes

Ingredients

- 4 ounces cream cheese, softened
- 1 teaspoon grated lemon zest
- 1 teaspoon Dijon mustard
- 2 tablespoons chopped scallions (white and green parts)
- Pink salt
- Freshly ground black pepper
- 1 (4-ounce) package cold-smoked salmon

Instructions

1. Combine the cream cheese, lemon zest, Dijon mustard, and scallions in a food processor or blender. Season with pink salt and pepper, then process until smooth.
2. Spread the cream cheese mixture evenly over each slice of salmon and roll tightly.
3. Arrange seam-side down on a plate and serve immediately, or refrigerate for up to 3 days.

Substitution Tip
Fresh dill or capers may be used in place of scallions.

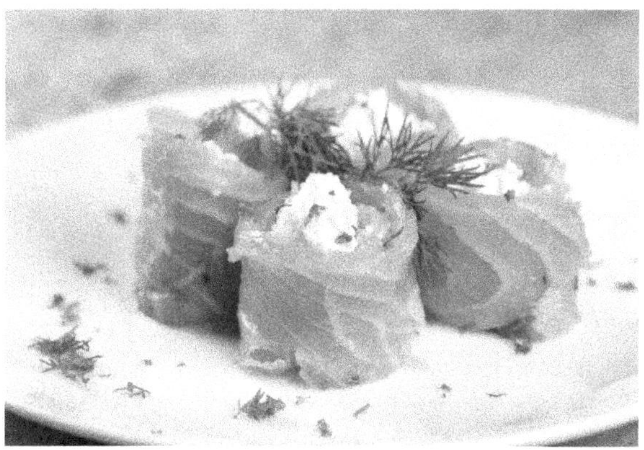

BRUSSELS SPROUTS, BACON & EGGS

Brussels sprouts may not be a traditional breakfast ingredient, but once you try them this way, you may never look back. Roasted with bacon and baked eggs, this dish is wholesome, flavorful, and incredibly easy to prepare.

30-MINUTE
Serves: 2
Prep: 5 minutes
Cook: 20 minutes

Instructions

1. Preheat the oven to 400°F (205°C).
2. Toss the Brussels sprouts with olive oil, pink salt, and black pepper.
3. Spray a 9×13-inch baking dish with nonstick spray.
4. Add the Brussels sprouts and diced bacon, then roast for 12 minutes.
5. Remove from the oven, stir, and create four wells in the mixture.
6. Crack one egg into each well.
7. Season with salt, pepper, and red pepper flakes.
8. Sprinkle Parmesan cheese over the top.
9. Return to the oven and bake for 8 minutes, or until the eggs reach your desired doneness.

Substitution Tip
Omit the Parmesan and use chopped salted nuts for a dairy-free option.

BLT BREAKFAST SALAD

Salads aren't just for lunch or dinner. A hearty breakfast salad is quick, nourishing, and incredibly satisfying—especially when topped with a soft-boiled egg, creamy avocado, and crispy bacon.

30-MINUTE
Serves: 2
Prep: 10 minutes
Cook: 5 minutes

Instructions

1. Bring a small saucepan of water to a boil. Gently add the eggs, reduce heat slightly, and cook for about 6 minutes.
2. While the eggs cook, toss the mixed greens with olive oil, salt, and pepper. Divide between two bowls.
3. Top with avocado slices, tomatoes, and bacon.
4. Peel and halve the eggs, place them on the salads, season lightly, and serve.

Substitution Tip
Fresh spinach or massaged kale makes an excellent alternative base.

CHEESY EGG & SPINACH NEST

This dish is as simple as it is impressive. Crispy melted cheese forms a nest around sunny-side-up eggs, creating a beautiful contrast of textures and flavors.

30-MINUTE • ONE PAN • VEGETARIAN
Serves: 1

Instructions

1. Heat olive oil in a skillet over medium-high heat.
2. Crack the eggs into the pan, close together, and season.
3. Once the whites begin to set, sprinkle mozzarella around the perimeter of the eggs.
4. Add the avocado and spinach to the cheese nest.
5. Sprinkle Parmesan over the top.
6. Cook until the cheese edges are golden and crisp.
7. Transfer to a warm plate and serve immediately.

Substitution Tip
Fresh flat-leaf parsley may replace spinach.

KALE–AVOCADO EGG SKILLET

This hearty one-skillet breakfast combines mushrooms, kale, eggs, and avocado for a nourishing, low-carb start to the day.

30-MINUTE • VEGETARIAN
Serves: 2

Instructions

1. Heat 1 tablespoon olive oil in a skillet and sauté mushrooms for about 3 minutes.
2. Massage kale with the remaining olive oil, then add to the skillet. Top with avocado slices.
3. Create four wells and crack one egg into each.
4. Season, cover, and cook for about 5 minutes, or until eggs are done to preference.
5. Serve hot.

Substitution Tip
Asparagus, tomatoes, or other keto-friendly vegetables work well here.

EGG-IN-A-HOLE BREAKFAST BURGER

Breakfast burgers are fun, indulgent, and deeply satisfying. A gooey egg, crispy bacon, melted cheese, and a juicy beef patty make this a standout morning meal.

30-MINUTE • ONE PAN
Serves: 2

Instructions

1. Cook bacon until crisp and set aside.
2. Form ground beef into patties and cut a hole in the center of each.
3. Melt butter in the skillet and cook patties for 2 minutes per side.
4. Crack an egg into each center and cook until whites set.
5. Top with Cheddar, cover to melt, then serve with bacon and Sriracha mayo.

PANCAKE "CAKE"

Love pancakes but hate standing over the stove flipping batch after batch? This recipe is for you. Using my Cream Cheese and Coconut Flour Pancake batter, this oven-baked version delivers all the flavor with none of the fuss. The result is a light, fluffy pancake "cake" that's perfect for slicing and serving family-style. Top it with butter, low-carb syrup, or your favorite keto-friendly additions. For extra flavor ideas, see the Variations.

30-MINUTE • VEGETARIAN
SERVES: 4
PREP: 5 minutes
COOK: 20 minutes

Ingredients

- 4 tablespoons butter, plus more for greasing the pan and topping

- 8 large eggs

- 8 ounces cream cheese, at room temperature

- 4 teaspoons liquid stevia

- 3 teaspoons baking powder

- ½ cup coconut flour

Instructions

1. Preheat the oven to 425°F. Generously butter a 9 × 13-inch baking pan.

2. In a food processor or blender, combine the eggs, cream cheese, stevia, baking powder, and coconut flour. Blend until smooth and fully incorporated.

3. Stir in any optional add-ins (see Variations), if using.

4. Spread the 4 tablespoons of butter evenly across the prepared pan.

5. Place the pan in the oven for 2–3 minutes, just until the butter melts and begins to bubble. Do not allow it to brown. Remove from the oven.

6. Pour the batter evenly into the pan.

7. Bake for about 15 minutes, or until a knife inserted into the center comes out clean.

8. Transfer the pan to a cooling rack and, if desired, melt a little extra butter over the top.

9. Slice into four portions and serve warm.

Ingredient Tip: I always add 2 teaspoons of vanilla extract and 2 teaspoons of ground cinnamon to the batter—it never disappoints.

Per Batch:
Calories: 2009 | Fat: 172g | Carbs: 51g | Net Carbs: 31g | Fiber: 20g | Protein: 72g

Per Serving:
Calories: 502 | Fat: 43g | Carbs: 13g | Net Carbs: 8g | Fiber: 5g | Protein: 18g

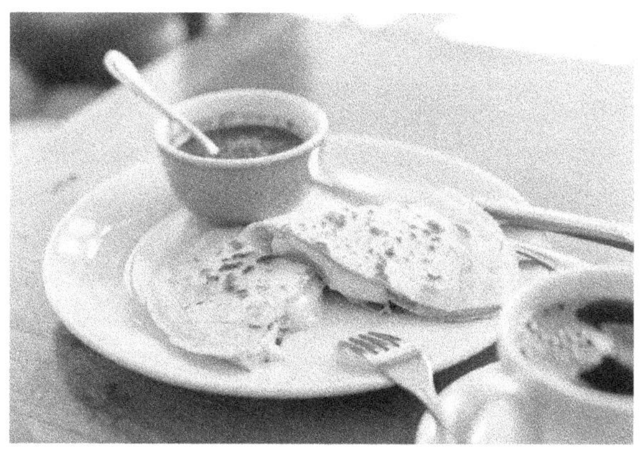

BREAKFAST QUESADILLA

Breakfast quesadillas are a favorite in my home—especially with my daughter. If she had her way, she'd eat them daily, but I usually make them once a week to keep them special. While scrambled eggs work well, I prefer fried eggs for the rich, gooey yolk that melts beautifully into the filling. For this recipe, I use Mission Whole Wheat Low-Carb Tortillas, which contain just 4 net carbs per tortilla.

30-MINUTE • ONE PAN
SERVES: 2
PREP: 5 minutes
COOK: 20 minutes

Ingredients
- 2 slices bacon

- 2 large eggs

- Pink salt

- Freshly ground black pepper

- 1 tablespoon olive oil

- 2 low-carbohydrate tortillas

- 1 cup shredded Mexican-blend cheese, divided

- ½ avocado, thinly sliced

Instructions

1. Heat a medium skillet over medium-high heat and cook the bacon until crispy, about 8 minutes, turning once. Transfer to a paper towel–lined plate and allow to cool slightly, then chop.

2. Reduce the heat to medium and crack the eggs into the skillet with the bacon grease. Season with pink salt and black pepper.

3. Cook for 3–4 minutes, until the whites are set. Cook longer if you prefer firm yolks. Transfer the eggs to a plate.

4. Add the olive oil to the skillet and place one tortilla in the pan.

5. Sprinkle ½ cup of cheese evenly over the tortilla. Arrange the avocado slices in a circle on top, followed by the fried eggs, chopped bacon, and remaining cheese. Cover with the second tortilla.

6. Once the cheese begins to melt and the bottom tortilla turns golden, about 3 minutes, carefully flip the quesadilla.

7. Cook the second side for another 2 minutes, until golden and crisp.

8. Slice with a pizza cutter or sharp knife and serve immediately.

Substitution Tip: Tajín seasoning can be used in place of salt and pepper for a bold blend of chili, lime, and salt.

Per Batch:
Calories: 1138 | Fat: 82g | Carbs: 53g | Net Carbs: 18g | Fiber: 35g | Protein: 54g

Per Serving:
Calories: 569 | Fat: 41g | Carbs: 27g | Net Carbs: 9g | Fiber: 18g | Protein: 27g

CREAM CHEESE MUFFINS

This recipe came together by happy accident. I planned to make sour-cream muffins but realized I was out, so I substituted cream cheese mixed with heavy whipping cream instead. The result was so rich and delicious that these muffins quickly became a regular favorite.

30-MINUTE • VEGETARIAN
MAKES: 6 muffins
PREP: 10 minutes
COOK: 10–12 minutes

Ingredients

- 4 tablespoons melted butter, plus more for greasing

- 1 cup almond flour

- ¾ tablespoon baking powder

- 2 large eggs, lightly beaten

- 2 ounces cream cheese mixed with 2 tablespoons heavy whipping cream

- A handful of shredded Mexican-blend cheese

Instructions

1. Preheat the oven to 400°F. Butter six cups of a muffin tin.

2. In a small bowl, whisk together the almond flour and baking powder.

3. In a medium bowl, combine the eggs, cream cheese mixture, shredded cheese, and melted butter.

4. Add the dry ingredients to the wet mixture and beat with a hand mixer until smooth.

5. Divide the batter evenly among the prepared muffin cups.

6. Bake for 12 minutes, or until the tops are golden. Serve warm.

Variations

This muffin batter is an excellent base for both savory and sweet options:

- Sprinkle *Everything But the Bagel* seasoning on top before baking for added crunch and flavor.

- Add diced jalapeños for a spicy kick.

- Stir in lemon zest and a handful of blueberries for a lightly sweet version.

Substitution Tip: Almond meal may be used instead of almond flour, though the texture will be slightly coarser.

Per Batch:
Calories: 1483 | Fat: 139g | Carbs: 34g | Net Carbs: 22g | Fiber: 12g | Protein: 45g

Per Serving:
Calories: 247 | Fat: 23g | Carbs: 6g | Net Carbs: 4g | Fiber: 2g | Protein: 8g

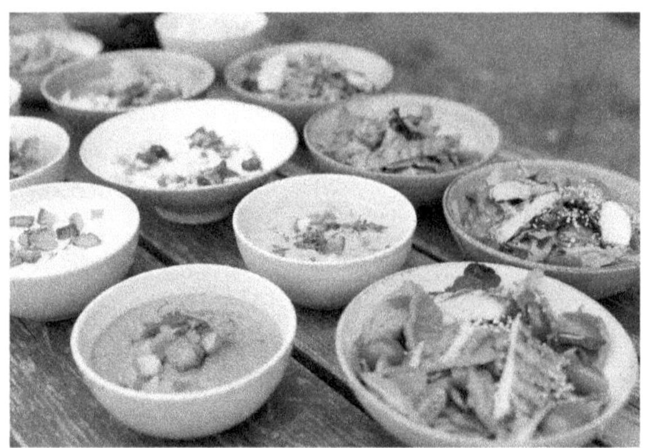

CHAPTER 3
HEARTY SOUPS & SALADS

Salads can be one of your greatest allies on a ketogenic diet—you just need to know what to watch out for. Many restaurant salads are packed with hidden sugars. Sometimes the sugar comes from high-carb fruits or dried fruits; other times it sneaks in through sweet dressings or candied nuts. To keep your salads keto-friendly, stick to the essentials: plenty of leafy greens, healthy fats, low-carb vegetables, high-fat nuts, and low-carb dressings. These five components ensure your salads are both flavorful and nutritionally balanced.

Soups are just as versatile for the keto lifestyle. If you're craving something hearty and filling, opt for cream-based, cheese-based, or cauliflower-based soups. These options deliver comfort and richness without unnecessary carbohydrates. One standout favorite in this chapter is the Creamy Tomato-Basil Soup—a recipe I've been making since "BK" (before keto). It remains one of my all-time favorites: simple, comforting, and incredibly delicious.

Recipes in This Chapter Include:
- Creamy Tomato-Basil Soup

- Broccoli-Cheese Soup

- Cheesy Cauliflower Soup

- Taco Soup

- Coconut and Cauliflower Curry Shrimp Soup

- Roasted Brussels Sprouts Salad with Parmesan

- BLT Wedge Salad

- Mexican Egg Salad

- Blue Cheese and Bacon Kale Salad

- Chopped Greek Salad

- Mediterranean Cucumber Salad

- Avocado Egg Salad Lettuce Cups

- Avocado Caprese Salad

- Shrimp and Avocado Salad

- Salmon Caesar Salad

- Salmon and Spinach Cobb Salad

- Taco Salad

- Cheeseburger Salad

- California Steak Salad

- Skirt Steak Cobb Salad

CREAMY TOMATO-BASIL SOUP

My parents always request this soup whenever I visit them. It's so fresh and creamy that once you make it, you'll never want canned tomato soup again.

30-MINUTE • VEGETARIAN
SERVES: 4
PREP: 5 minutes
COOK: 15 minutes

Ingredients

- 1 (14.5-ounce) can diced tomatoes (I use Muir Glen Organic Tomatoes with Italian Seasonings)

- 2 ounces cream cheese

- ¼ cup heavy (whipping) cream

- 4 tablespoons butter

- ¼ cup fresh basil leaves, chopped

- Pink salt

- Freshly ground black pepper

Instructions

1. Add the tomatoes with their juices to a food processor or blender and purée until smooth.

2. In a medium saucepan over medium heat, combine the puréed tomatoes, cream cheese, heavy cream, and butter. Cook for 10 minutes, stirring occasionally, until melted and fully combined.

3. Stir in the basil and season with pink salt and black pepper. Continue cooking for 5 minutes, stirring until completely smooth. An immersion blender may be used for an extra-silky texture.

4. Ladle into bowls and serve hot.

Ingredient Tip: Plain diced tomatoes work fine, but Italian-seasoned tomatoes add extra depth of flavor.

Per Serving:
Calories: 239 | Fat: 22g | Carbs: 9g | Net Carbs: 7g | Fiber: 2g | Protein: 3g

BROCCOLI-CHEESE SOUP

When the temperature drops below 60°F in Los Angeles, I instantly crave a hearty soup. This Broccoli-Cheese Soup is keto-perfect, satisfying, and flavorful enough to serve as a complete meal.

30-MINUTE • ONE POT • VEGETARIAN
SERVES: 4
PREP: 5 minutes
COOK: 20 minutes

Ingredients

- 2 tablespoons butter

- 1 cup broccoli florets, finely chopped

- 1 cup heavy (whipping) cream

- 1 cup chicken or vegetable broth

- Pink salt

- Freshly ground black pepper

- 1 cup shredded sharp Cheddar cheese, divided

Instructions

1. Melt the butter in a medium saucepan over medium heat.

2. Add the broccoli and sauté for about 5 minutes, until tender.

3. Stir in the cream and broth. Season with salt and pepper and cook for 10–15 minutes, stirring occasionally, until thickened.

4. Reduce heat to low and slowly add the cheese, stirring constantly. Reserve a small amount for topping.

5. Serve hot, topped with the reserved cheese.

Variations

- Add ¼ teaspoon red pepper flakes for heat.

- Add minced garlic and diced onion with the broccoli for deeper flavor.

- Top with crumbled bacon for a smoky crunch.

Ingredient Tip: For a smoother soup, blend before adding the cheese.

CHEESY CAULIFLOWER SOUP

Cauliflower proves once again that it can do it all. This soup is a keto-friendly twist on classic potato soup—rich, creamy, and completely satisfying without the carbs.

30-MINUTE • ONE POT
SERVES: 4

Instructions Summary
Sauté onion in butter, simmer cauliflower in broth until tender, mash and blend with cream cheese and heavy cream, then season and top with Cheddar cheese.

Variation Tip: Add bacon, scallions, or hot sauce for texture and heat.

TACO SOUP

This creamy, slow-cooked soup delivers bold taco flavor with minimal effort. Browning the beef beforehand adds extra depth, making this a rich and comforting keto favorite.

SLOW COOKER • SERVES 4

Ingredient Tip: Swap ground beef for spicy sausage for a flavor twist.

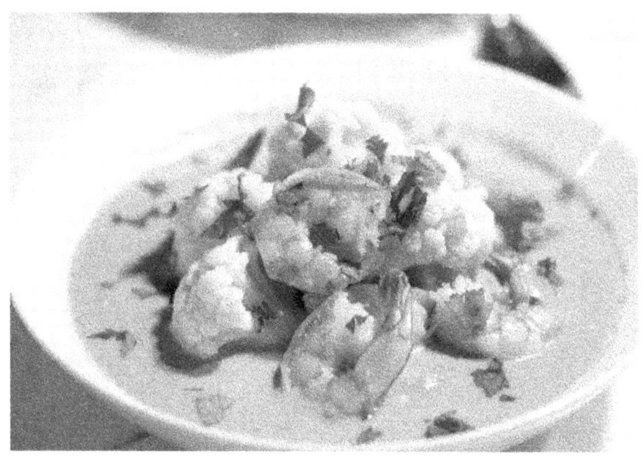

COCONUT AND CAULIFLOWER CURRY SHRIMP SOUP

This soup brings together spicy red curry, rich coconut milk, tender shrimp, and fresh cilantro for a perfectly balanced dish inspired by Asian flavors.

ONE POT • SLOW COOKER • SERVES 4

Ingredient Tip: Cooked, shredded chicken breast makes a great substitute for shrimp.

ROASTED BRUSSELS SPROUTS SALAD WITH PARMESAN

Unlike most roasted Brussels sprouts dishes, this salad uses only the leaves of the sprouts, resulting in a lighter, crispier texture. The roasted leaves pair beautifully with nutty Parmesan and crunchy hazelnuts, which truly shine in this simple but elegant salad.

30-MINUTE • VEGETARIAN

Serves: 2
Prep Time: 10 minutes
Cook Time: 15 minutes

Ingredients
- 1 pound Brussels sprouts

- 1 tablespoon olive oil

- Pink salt

- Freshly ground black pepper

- ¼ cup shaved or grated Parmesan cheese

- ¼ cup whole, skinless hazelnuts

Instructions
1. Preheat the oven to **350°F (180°C)**. Line a baking sheet with parchment paper or a silicone baking mat to prevent sticking and ensure even browning.

2. Using a small knife, trim off the stem end and core of each Brussels sprout. This will allow the leaves to naturally fall apart. Set the cores aside if you'd like to roast them later.

3. Place all the loose Brussels sprout leaves into a medium bowl. Use your hands to gently separate any remaining layers.

4. Drizzle the olive oil over the leaves, then season lightly with pink salt and freshly ground black pepper. Toss well to coat every leaf evenly.

5. Spread the leaves in a single, even layer on the prepared baking sheet. Avoid overcrowding so they roast rather than steam.

6. Roast for **10 to 15 minutes**, stirring once halfway through, until the leaves are lightly browned and crisp around the edges.

7. Divide the roasted Brussels sprout leaves between two bowls. Top each serving with Parmesan cheese and hazelnuts. Serve immediately while warm and crisp.

Substitution Tip: If hazelnuts aren't available, chopped almonds work well and offer a similar crunch.

BLT WEDGE SALAD

A crisp iceberg lettuce wedge is delicious on its own, but when topped with smoky bacon, juicy tomatoes, and rich blue cheese dressing, it becomes a satisfying and classic low-carb favorite.

30-MINUTE • ONE PAN

Serves: 2
Prep Time: 10 minutes
Cook Time: 10 minutes

Ingredients
- 4 bacon slices
- ½ head iceberg lettuce, cut into halves
- 2 tablespoons blue cheese dressing
- ¼ cup blue cheese crumbles
- ½ cup grape tomatoes, halved

Instructions
1. Heat a large skillet over medium-high heat. Add the bacon slices and cook for about **8 minutes**, turning occasionally, until crispy and evenly browned.

2. Transfer the cooked bacon to a paper towel–lined plate and allow it to cool for about **5 minutes**, then chop into bite-size pieces.

3. Place one lettuce wedge on each serving plate, positioning them cut-side up for easy topping.

4. Spoon half of the blue cheese dressing over each wedge.

5. Evenly distribute the blue cheese crumbles, halved tomatoes, and chopped bacon over the lettuce.

6. Serve immediately while the bacon is still warm and crisp.

Ingredient Tip: For a smoky twist, lightly grill the lettuce wedges for about **1 minute per side** after brushing with olive oil and seasoning with salt and pepper. Dress as directed after grilling.

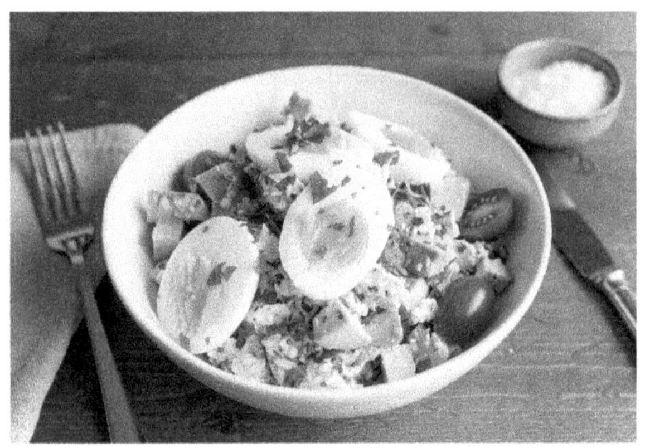

MEXICAN EGG SALAD

This bold twist on classic egg salad features creamy avocado, fresh cilantro, and jalapeño for heat. Serving it atop crispy cheese chips adds crunch and makes this dish extra satisfying.

30-MINUTE • VEGETARIAN

Serves: 2
Prep Time: 15 minutes
Cook Time: 10 minutes

Ingredients
For the Hard-Boiled Eggs

- 4 large eggs

For the Cheese Chips

- ½ cup shredded cheese (Mexican blend), divided

For the Mexican Egg Salad

- 1 jalapeño

- 1 avocado, halved

- Pink salt

- Freshly ground black pepper

- 2 tablespoons chopped fresh cilantro

Instructions
Make the Hard-Boiled Eggs
1. Place the eggs in a medium saucepan and cover completely with water.

2. Bring the water to a rolling boil over high heat. Once boiling, turn off the heat, cover the pan, and let the eggs sit for **10 to 12 minutes**.

3. Transfer the eggs to cold running water or an ice bath for **1 minute** to stop the cooking.

4. Gently crack and peel the eggs. Set aside.

Make the Cheese Chips
1. Preheat the oven to **350°F (180°C)** and line a baking sheet with parchment paper.

2. Place two equal mounds (¼ cup each) of shredded cheese on the baking sheet, spacing them well apart.

3. Bake for **7 minutes**, or until the cheese is fully melted and the edges are lightly browned.

4. Remove from the oven and let cool for **5 minutes**. The chips will firm up as they cool.

Make the Egg Salad
1. Chop the peeled hard-boiled eggs and place them in a medium bowl.

2. Remove the stem, ribs, and seeds from the jalapeño, then finely dice and add to the bowl.

3. Mash the avocado with a fork until mostly smooth. Season with pink salt and black pepper.

4. Add the mashed avocado and chopped cilantro to the eggs and gently stir until well combined.

5. Place one cheese chip on each plate, top with the egg salad, and serve immediately.

BLUE CHEESE AND BACON KALE SALAD

Massaging kale with dressing softens its fibers, making it tender and easier to digest. Paired with crispy bacon, blue cheese, and pecans, this salad delivers rich flavor and texture in every bite.

30-MINUTE

Serves: 2
Prep Time: 10 minutes
Cook Time: 10 minutes

Ingredients
- 4 bacon slices

- 2 cups fresh kale, stemmed and chopped

- 1 tablespoon vinaigrette dressing

- Pinch pink salt

- Pinch freshly ground black pepper

- ¼ cup pecans

- ¼ cup blue cheese crumbles

Instructions
1. Cook the bacon in a medium skillet over medium-high heat for about **8 minutes**, turning occasionally, until crisp.

2. Transfer the bacon to a paper towel–lined plate to drain.

3. Place the chopped kale in a large bowl. Add the vinaigrette and massage the kale with clean hands for **2 minutes**, until it becomes darker and softer.

4. Season the kale with pink salt and black pepper, then let it rest while the bacon cools.

5. Chop the bacon and pecans, then add them to the bowl along with the blue cheese crumbles.

6. Toss well to combine, divide between two plates, and serve.

Substitution Tip: Chopped almonds can be used in place of pecans.

CHOPPED GREEK SALAD

Fresh, crisp, and endlessly customizable, this chopped Greek salad comes together quickly and makes a perfect light meal or side dish.

30-MINUTE • ONE POT • NO COOK • VEGETARIAN

Serves: 2
Prep Time: 10 minutes

Ingredients
- 2 cups chopped romaine lettuce

- ½ cup grape tomatoes, halved

- ¼ cup sliced black olives

- ¼ cup feta cheese crumbles

- 2 tablespoons vinaigrette dressing

- Pink salt

- Freshly ground black pepper

- 1 tablespoon olive oil

Instructions
1. Place the romaine, tomatoes, olives, feta cheese, and vinaigrette into a large bowl.

2. Season lightly with pink salt and freshly ground black pepper.

3. Drizzle with olive oil and toss gently until all ingredients are evenly coated.

4. Divide the salad between two bowls and serve immediately.

Variations

- Add chopped cucumbers, red onion, or pepperoncini for extra crunch and brightness.

- For a heartier version, mix in finely chopped Genoa salami or pepperoni.

Substitution Tip: Goat cheese can be used in place of feta.

MEDITERRANEAN CUCUMBER SALAD

This refreshing salad is simple, vibrant, and full of Mediterranean flavor. Crisp cucumbers and juicy tomatoes bring freshness, while olives and feta add satisfying healthy fats. It's an ideal side dish for grilled or roasted Mediterranean-style meats.

30-MINUTE • ONE POT • VEGETARIAN

Serves: 2
Prep Time: 10 minutes

Ingredients
- 1 large cucumber, peeled and finely chopped

- ½ cup grape tomatoes, halved

- ¼ cup black olives, halved

- ¼ cup crumbled feta cheese

- Pink salt

- Freshly ground black pepper

- 2 tablespoons vinaigrette dressing

Instructions
1. Place the chopped cucumber, halved tomatoes, olives, and feta cheese into a large mixing bowl.

2. Season lightly with pink salt and freshly ground black pepper.

3. Drizzle the vinaigrette over the salad.

4. Toss gently until all ingredients are evenly coated with dressing.

5. Divide the salad between two bowls and serve immediately.

Ingredient Tip: This salad tastes great right away, but for deeper flavor, cover and refrigerate for a few hours to allow the dressing to marinate the vegetables.

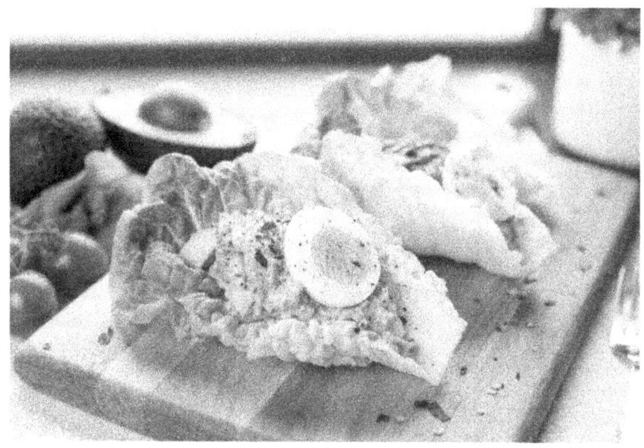

AVOCADO EGG SALAD LETTUCE CUPS

Replacing mayonnaise with avocado gives this egg salad a creamy texture and fresh flavor. Served in crisp lettuce cups and topped with sliced radishes, it's light, crunchy, and incredibly satisfying.

30-MINUTE • VEGETARIAN

Serves: 2
Prep Time: 15 minutes
Cook Time: 15 minutes

Ingredients
For the Hard-Boiled Eggs

- 4 large eggs

For the Egg Salad

- 1 avocado, halved

- Pink salt

- Freshly ground black pepper

- ½ teaspoon freshly squeezed lemon juice

- 4 butter lettuce cups, washed and dried

- 2 radishes, thinly sliced

Instructions
Make the Hard-Boiled Eggs
1. Place the eggs in a medium saucepan and cover with water.

2. Bring the water to a rolling boil over high heat.

3. Once boiling, turn off the heat, cover the pan, and let the eggs sit on the hot burner for **10–12 minutes**.

4. Transfer the eggs to cold running water or an ice bath for **1 minute**.

5. Gently tap and peel the eggs. Set aside.

Make the Egg Salad
1. Chop the peeled eggs and place them in a medium bowl.

2. Add the avocado flesh and mash gently with a fork.

3. Season with pink salt, black pepper, and lemon juice.

4. Stir until the mixture is creamy but still slightly chunky.

5. Arrange the lettuce cups on two plates.

6. Spoon the egg salad into the cups and top with sliced radishes.

7. Serve immediately.

Variations

- Add diced jalapeño and red onion for a guacamole-style twist.

- Add chopped or sliced crispy bacon for extra crunch.

Substitution Tip: Romaine hearts or baby cos lettuce work well if butter lettuce isn't available.

AVOCADO CAPRESE SALAD

This keto-friendly take on a classic Caprese salad adds avocado for richness and arugula for a peppery bite. The result is a filling, flavorful dish that's perfect as a light meal or side.

30-MINUTE • NO COOK • VEGETARIAN

Serves: 2
Prep Time: 5 minutes

Ingredients
- 2 cups arugula
- 1 tablespoon olive oil, divided
- Pink salt
- Freshly ground black pepper
- 1 avocado, sliced
- 4 fresh mozzarella balls, sliced
- 1 Roma tomato, sliced
- 4 fresh basil leaves, thinly sliced

Instructions
1. Place the arugula in a large bowl.
2. Drizzle with ½ tablespoon of olive oil and season lightly with pink salt and pepper.
3. Toss gently until the arugula is evenly coated.
4. Divide the arugula between two plates.

5. Arrange the avocado, mozzarella, and tomato slices evenly over the greens.

6. Drizzle with the remaining olive oil and season again lightly with salt and pepper.

7. Sprinkle with fresh basil and serve.

Substitution Tip: For extra flavor, replace the olive oil with a vinaigrette dressing.

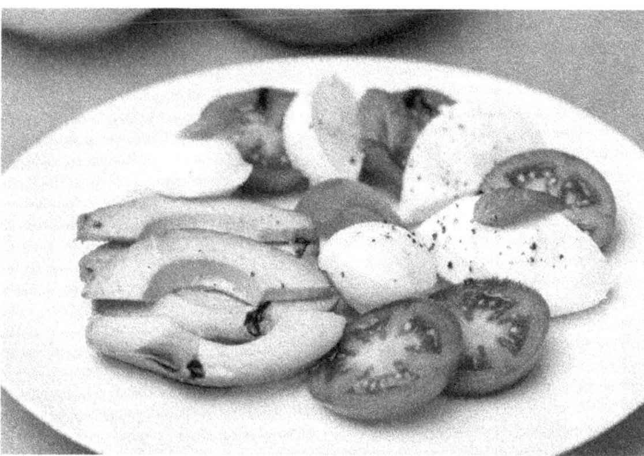

SHRIMP AND AVOCADO SALAD

This chilled salad is creamy, refreshing, and worth the short wait before serving. Using pre-cooked shrimp makes it quick and effortless.

Serves: 2
Prep Time: 5 minutes, plus 30 minutes chilling
Cook Time: 2 minutes

Ingredients

- 1 tablespoon olive oil

- 1 pound cooked shrimp, peeled and deveined

- Pink salt

- Freshly ground black pepper

- 1 avocado, cubed

- 1 celery stalk, chopped

- ¼ cup mayonnaise

- 1 teaspoon freshly squeezed lime juice

Instructions

1. Heat the olive oil in a large skillet over medium heat.

2. Add the shrimp and cook for **1–2 minutes**, just until warmed through and pink.

3. Season lightly with pink salt and pepper.

4. Transfer the shrimp to a bowl, cover, and refrigerate to cool.

5. In a separate bowl, combine the avocado, celery, mayonnaise, and lime juice.

6. Season lightly with pink salt and stir until creamy.

7. Add the chilled shrimp and toss gently to combine.

8. Cover and refrigerate for **30 minutes** before serving.

Variations

- Add chopped fresh dill for brightness.

- Serve the salad in butter lettuce or romaine leaves for added crunch.

Substitution Tip: Use Tajín seasoning instead of salt for a citrusy kick.

SALMON CAESAR SALAD

This rich and satisfying salad replaces croutons with crispy bacon for crunch. Creamy Caesar dressing pairs beautifully with pan-seared salmon.

30-MINUTE • ONE PAN

Serves: 2
Prep Time: 5 minutes
Cook Time: 20 minutes

Instructions
1. Cook the bacon in a skillet over medium-high heat until crispy, about **8 minutes**. Transfer to a paper towel–lined plate.

2. Pat the salmon fillets dry and season both sides with pink salt and pepper.

3. Using the bacon grease in the skillet, add the salmon. Add ghee if needed.

4. Cook the salmon for **5 minutes per side**, or until desired doneness.

5. Tear the bacon into pieces.

6. Divide the romaine, avocado slices, and bacon between two plates.

7. Top each salad with a salmon fillet.

8. Drizzle with Caesar dressing and serve.

SALMON AND SPINACH COBB SALAD

This keto-friendly Cobb salad features salmon and soft-boiled eggs, with the warm yolk acting as a natural dressing.

30-MINUTE

Serves: 2
Prep Time: 5 minutes
Cook Time: 25 minutes

Instructions
1. Cook the bacon in a skillet until crispy and set aside.

2. Bring a small saucepan of water to a boil. Add the eggs and cook for **6 minutes** for soft-boiled.

3. Pat the salmon dry and season with salt and pepper.

4. Cook the salmon in the bacon grease, adding ghee if needed, for **5 minutes per side**.

5. Chop the bacon and peel the eggs.

6. Divide the spinach, avocado, and bacon between two plates.

7. Halve the eggs and place on top.

8. Sprinkle with blue cheese.

9. Top with salmon, drizzle with olive oil, and serve.

TACO SALAD

This easy taco salad skips the shell but keeps all the flavor, making it a perfect keto-friendly meal.

30-MINUTE • ONE PAN

Instructions
1. Heat ghee in a skillet over medium-high heat.

2. Add the ground beef, breaking it up as it cooks.

3. Brown for **10 minutes**, seasoning with salt and pepper.

4. Divide romaine into bowls and season lightly.

5. Top with avocado, tomatoes, beef, and cheese.

6. Serve immediately.

CHEESEBURGER SALAD

All the flavors of a lettuce-wrapped cheeseburger, tossed together in one bowl.

30-MINUTE

Instructions
1. Heat ghee in a skillet over medium-high heat.

2. Brown the ground beef for **10 minutes**, seasoning with salt and pepper.

3. Place pickles, romaine, and cheese in a large bowl.

4. Transfer beef using a slotted spoon.

5. Add dressing and toss thoroughly.

6. Divide and serve.

CALIFORNIA STEAK SALAD

Avocados and strawberries are a perfect match, bringing fresh and fruity notes that complement the peppery arugula and tender skirt steak beautifully. This vibrant salad bursts with California flavors.

30-MINUTE

Serves: 2
Prep Time: 15 minutes
Cook Time: 10 minutes

Ingredients
- 8 ounces skirt steak

- Pink salt

- Freshly ground black pepper

- 2 tablespoons butter

- 2 cups arugula

- 1 tablespoon olive oil

- 1 avocado, sliced

- 2 fresh strawberries, sliced

- ¼ cup slivered, chopped almonds

Instructions
1. Heat a large skillet over high heat until very hot.

2. Pat the skirt steak dry with paper towels to remove any moisture. This helps create a good sear.

3. Season both sides of the steak generously with pink salt and freshly ground black pepper.

4. Add the butter to the hot skillet. When the butter has melted and is sizzling, place the steak in the skillet.

5. Sear the steak for about **3 minutes on each side** to achieve medium-rare doneness. Adjust cooking time if you prefer it more or less done.

6. Remove the steak from the skillet and transfer it to a cutting board. Let it rest for **at least 5 minutes** to allow the juices to redistribute.

7. While the steak rests, place the arugula in a large bowl. Toss with olive oil, then season lightly with salt and pepper.

8. Divide the dressed arugula evenly between two plates.

9. Top the greens with sliced avocado, sliced strawberries, and slivered almonds.

10. Slice the rested steak thinly **against the grain** to maximize tenderness.

11. Arrange the sliced steak over the salads and serve immediately.

Substitution Tip: Flank steak works equally well here. For convenience, you can also use thinly sliced leftover cooked steak.

SKIRT STEAK COBB SALAD

Skirt steak is ideal for this salad because it cooks quickly and delivers rich flavor. Cook it medium-rare for tenderness, and slice across the grain when serving. No marinade is needed, but seasoning with salt and pepper and cooking on a very hot pan brings out the best taste.

30-MINUTE • ONE PAN

Serves: 2
Prep Time: 15 minutes
Cook Time: 10 minutes

Ingredients
- 8 ounces skirt steak
- Pink salt
- Freshly ground black pepper
- 1 tablespoon butter
- 2 romaine hearts or 2 cups chopped romaine lettuce
- ½ cup halved grape tomatoes
- ¼ cup crumbled blue cheese
- ¼ cup pecans
- 1 tablespoon olive oil

Instructions
1. Preheat a large skillet over high heat until it's very hot.
2. Pat the skirt steak dry with paper towels.

3. Season both sides of the steak with pink salt and black pepper.

4. Add butter to the skillet. When melted and sizzling, carefully place the steak in the pan.

5. Cook the steak for **about 3 minutes per side** for medium-rare, adjusting time to your preferred doneness.

6. Remove the steak from the pan and transfer it to a cutting board. Let it rest for **at least 5 minutes**.

7. Meanwhile, divide the romaine lettuce between two plates.

8. Top the lettuce with halved grape tomatoes, crumbled blue cheese, and pecans.

9. Drizzle the olive oil evenly over the salads.

10. Slice the rested steak thinly **against the grain**.

11. Arrange the sliced steak on top of each salad and serve.

Variations

Salads are a perfect base for your creativity! Here are some tasty ideas you can try:

- Add a drizzle of balsamic dressing and a sliced hard-boiled egg for extra richness.

- Substitute walnuts for pecans and add one sliced avocado for extra creaminess.

Substitution Tip: Flank steak is a great alternative to skirt steak here as well.

Nutritional Information

Recipe	Per Batch	Per Serving
California Steak Salad	Calories: 1001	Calories: 501
	Total Fat: 81g	Total Fat: 41g
	Carbs: 21g	Carbs: 11g
	Net Carbs: 8g	Net Carbs: 4g
	Fiber: 13g	Fiber: 7g
	Protein: 55g	Protein: 28g
Skirt Steak Cobb Salad	Calories: 902	Calories: 451
	Total Fat: 71g	Total Fat: 36g
	Carbs: 14g	Carbs: 7g
	Net Carbs: 9g	Net Carbs: 5g
	Fiber: 6g	Fiber: 3g
	Protein: 60g	Protein: 30g

CHAPTER 4
SIDE DISHES & SNACKS

These side dishes bring exciting flavors to your keto table. Often, I enjoy one of these veggie-forward recipes as my main meal when I'm craving something light and fresh, but they also pair beautifully alongside your favorite protein. This chapter highlights some of the many creative ways to enjoy vegetables on a keto diet.

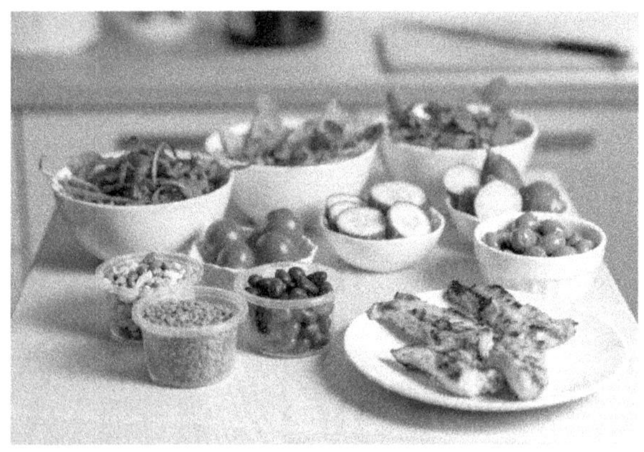

ROASTED CAULIFLOWER WITH PROSCIUTTO, CAPERS, AND ALMONDS

This is one of my all-time favorite dishes. I often eat it for dinner, but it also makes a fantastic side with any meat. The capers add a sharp, tangy pop of flavor, while the slivered almonds give a delightful crunch. I like roasting cauliflower right after cooking bacon to use that flavorful leftover bacon grease. Sometimes I even toss seasoned chicken breasts into the pan alongside the cauliflower for a complete one-pan meal.

30-MINUTE • ONE PAN
Serves: 2

Prep: 5 minutes
Cook: 25 minutes

Ingredients:

- 12 ounces cauliflower florets (precut works great)

- 2 tablespoons leftover bacon grease or olive oil

- Pink salt

- Freshly ground black pepper

- 2 ounces sliced prosciutto, torn into small pieces

- ¼ cup slivered almonds

- 2 tablespoons capers

- 2 tablespoons grated Parmesan cheese

Instructions:

1. Preheat your oven to 400°F. Line a baking pan with a silicone baking mat or parchment paper.

2. Place the cauliflower florets in the prepared pan. Drizzle with bacon grease or olive oil, then season with pink salt and freshly ground black pepper. Toss to coat evenly.

3. Roast the cauliflower for 15 minutes.

4. Remove the pan and stir the cauliflower to ensure all sides soak up the bacon grease.

5. Add the torn prosciutto, slivered almonds, and capers to the pan. Toss gently to combine. Sprinkle the Parmesan cheese evenly on top.

6. Return to the oven and roast for another 10 minutes until the cauliflower is tender and the almonds are toasted.

7. Using a slotted spoon, divide the cauliflower between two plates, leaving excess grease behind. Serve warm.

Substitution Tip: If you don't have capers, sliced green olives make a delicious alternative.

Nutrition (Per Serving):
Calories: 288 | Total Fat: 24g | Carbs: 7g | Net Carbs: 4g | Fiber: 3g | Protein: 14g

BUTTERY SLOW-COOKER MUSHROOMS

There's something magical about dry ranch-dressing mix that elevates these mushrooms with savory, comforting flavor. This slow-cooker recipe fills your house with an irresistible aroma. I love snacking on these while watching football, but they also make a rich and buttery side dish for many meats. You can easily double or triple this for a crowd.

ONE POT • VEGETARIAN
Serves: 2
Prep: 10 minutes
Cook: 4 hours

Ingredients:

- 6 tablespoons butter

- 1 tablespoon packaged dry ranch-dressing mix

- 8 ounces fresh cremini mushrooms

- 2 tablespoons grated Parmesan cheese

- 1 tablespoon chopped fresh flat-leaf Italian parsley

Instructions:

1. With the crock insert in place, preheat the slow cooker on low.

2. Add butter and dry ranch dressing mix to the slow cooker base. Stir occasionally until the butter melts and the mix is well blended.

3. Add the cremini mushrooms and stir to coat them thoroughly with the butter and ranch mixture. Sprinkle Parmesan cheese evenly over the top.

4. Cover and cook on low for 4 hours, allowing mushrooms to soften and soak up all the flavor.

5. Use a slotted spoon to transfer the mushrooms to a serving dish. Garnish with chopped parsley and serve.

Substitution Tip: If you don't have dry ranch mix, combine equal parts onion powder, garlic powder, dried thyme, pink salt, pepper, dried parsley, and a dash of paprika for a similar seasoning blend.

Nutrition (Per Serving):
Calories: 351 | Total Fat: 36g | Carbs: 5g | Net Carbs: 4g | Fiber: 1g | Protein: 6g

BAKED ZUCCHINI GRATIN

I love a classic gratin — but with potatoes off the table, this cheesy zucchini version with a crispy pork rind topping hits the spot perfectly. Crushed pork rinds add a crunchy, breadcrumb-like texture and you can use any flavor you prefer. The creamy mix of Brie and Gruyère cheeses makes this dish uniquely delicious.

Serves: 2
Prep: 10 minutes + 30 minutes draining
Cook: 25 minutes

Ingredients:

- 1 large zucchini, sliced into ¼-inch thick rounds

- Pink salt

- 1 ounce Brie cheese, rind removed

- 1 tablespoon butter

- Freshly ground black pepper

- ⅓ cup shredded Gruyère cheese

- ⅓ cup crushed pork rinds

Instructions:

1. Salt the zucchini slices generously and place them in a colander over the sink. Let them drain for about 45 minutes to release excess water.

2. Preheat the oven to 400°F.

3. While the zucchini drains, melt the Brie and butter together in a small saucepan over medium-low heat,

stirring occasionally until smooth and combined (about 2 minutes).

4. Arrange the zucchini slices in an 8-inch baking dish, overlapping slightly. Season with freshly ground black pepper.

5. Pour the melted Brie mixture evenly over the zucchini. Sprinkle shredded Gruyère cheese on top.

6. Finish by sprinkling the crushed pork rinds over the cheese layer.

7. Bake for about 25 minutes, until bubbly and golden brown on top. Serve warm.

Substitution Tip: Crème de Brie or other soft Brie-style cheeses with garlic or herbs can add an extra flavor boost.

Nutrition (Per Serving):
Calories: 355 | Total Fat: 25g | Carbs: 5g | Net Carbs: 4g | Fiber: 2g | Protein: 28g

ROASTED RADISHES WITH BROWN BUTTER SAUCE

These warm roasted radishes have the crispy exterior and creamy interior of baby red potatoes but are much lower in carbs. The nutty brown butter sauce takes this dish to a new level of deliciousness.

30-MINUTE • VEGETARIAN
Serves: 2
Prep: 10 minutes
Cook: 15 minutes

Ingredients:

- 2 cups halved radishes
- 1 tablespoon olive oil
- Pink salt
- Freshly ground black pepper
- 2 tablespoons butter
- 1 tablespoon chopped fresh flat-leaf Italian parsley

Instructions:

1. Preheat the oven to 450°F.

2. Toss the halved radishes with olive oil, then season with pink salt and freshly ground black pepper.

3. Spread the radishes evenly on a baking sheet and roast for 15 minutes, stirring once halfway through.

4. When the radishes have about 5 minutes left to roast, melt the butter in a small light-colored

saucepan over medium heat. Stir frequently and season with pink salt.

5. Continue cooking the butter until it foams and bubbles, then the bubbling slows and the butter turns a rich nutty brown, about 3 minutes. Remove from heat and transfer to a heat-safe container.

6. Once radishes are done, divide them between two plates and spoon the brown butter sauce over the top. Garnish with chopped parsley and serve immediately.

Ingredient Tip: Feel free to roast radishes with their stems on for a rustic look and added flavor.

Nutrition (Per Serving):
Calories: 181 | Total Fat: 19g | Carbs: 4g | Net Carbs: 2g | Fiber: 2g | Protein: 1g

PARMESAN AND PORK RIND GREEN BEANS

I adore green beans, and roasting them has quickly become my favorite way to cook most vegetables. Coated in olive oil, Parmesan cheese, and crushed pork rinds, these green beans are bursting with flavor and texture.

30-MINUTE
Serves: 2
Prep: 5 minutes
Cook: 15 minutes

Ingredients:

- ½ pound fresh green beans

- 2 tablespoons crushed pork rinds

- 2 tablespoons olive oil

- 1 tablespoon grated Parmesan cheese

- Pink salt

- Freshly ground black pepper

Instructions:

1. Preheat the oven to 400°F.

2. In a medium bowl, toss the green beans with crushed pork rinds, olive oil, Parmesan cheese, pink salt, and pepper until evenly coated.

3. Spread the mixture in a single layer on a baking sheet.

4. Roast for about 15 minutes, stirring or shaking the pan halfway through to ensure even cooking.

5. Divide the green beans between two plates and serve.

Ingredient Tip: Use any flavored pork rinds you like for a different twist — I usually stick to the original flavor.

Nutrition (Per Serving):
Calories: 175 | Total Fat: 15g | Carbs: 8g | Net Carbs: 5g | Fiber: 3g | Protein: 6g

PESTO CAULIFLOWER STEAKS

I love making pesto whenever I buy fresh basil—any leftover bunches turn into this vibrant sauce. I usually use whatever nuts I have on hand; almonds are my favorite. The rich, flavorful pesto paired with melted cheese is the perfect topping for roasted cauliflower steaks.

30-MINUTE • VEGETARIAN
Serves: 2
Prep: 5 minutes
Cook: 20 minutes

Ingredients:
- 2 tablespoons olive oil, plus extra for brushing
- ½ head cauliflower
- Pink salt
- Freshly ground black pepper
- 2 cups fresh basil leaves
- ½ cup grated Parmesan cheese
- ¼ cup almonds
- ½ cup shredded mozzarella cheese

Instructions:
1. Preheat the oven to 425°F. Lightly brush a baking sheet with olive oil or line it with a silicone baking mat.

2. Remove the leaves from the cauliflower and slice it into 1-inch-thick "steaks." Don't discard the smaller florets that fall off—roast them alongside the steaks.

3. Place the cauliflower steaks on the prepared baking sheet. Brush lightly with olive oil to encourage caramelization. Season with pink salt and freshly ground black pepper.

4. Roast the cauliflower steaks for 20 minutes, until tender and golden.

5. While the cauliflower roasts, combine the basil, Parmesan cheese, almonds, and 2 tablespoons olive oil in a food processor or blender. Season with pink salt and pepper, then blend until smooth to create the pesto.

6. Spread a generous amount of pesto on each cauliflower steak, then top with shredded mozzarella cheese. Return to the oven and bake for another 2 minutes, or until the cheese melts.

7. Serve the cauliflower steaks hot on plates, enjoying the rich layers of flavor.

Substitution Tip: I prefer almonds for pesto instead of pine nuts simply because I always have almonds on hand. But pine nuts work just as well if you have them.

TOMATO, AVOCADO, AND CUCUMBER SALAD

This quick and fresh salad comes together in minutes, making it a perfect dish for potlucks or light meals. I recommend using small Persian cucumbers for their crisp texture and tiny seeds.

30-MINUTE • NO COOK • VEGETARIAN
Serves: 2
Prep: 5 minutes

Ingredients:

- ½ cup grape tomatoes, halved

- 4 small Persian cucumbers, or 1 English cucumber, peeled and finely chopped

- 1 avocado, finely chopped

- ¼ cup crumbled feta cheese

- 2 tablespoons vinaigrette salad dressing (I like Primal Kitchen Greek Vinaigrette)

- Pink salt

- Freshly ground black pepper

Instructions:

1. In a large bowl, combine the halved tomatoes, chopped cucumbers, avocado, and crumbled feta cheese.

2. Add the vinaigrette dressing, then season with pink salt and freshly ground black pepper. Toss gently to combine all ingredients evenly.

3. Divide the salad onto two plates and serve immediately.

Variations:

- Add ½ finely chopped red onion for extra crunch and freshness.

- Include sliced black olives for a briny twist.

Substitution Tip: Goat cheese can be swapped in place of feta for a creamier texture and tangier flavor.

CRUNCHY PORK RIND ZUCCHINI STICKS

My daughter isn't usually a fan of zucchini, but she absolutely loves these crunchy, salty zucchini sticks. They make a delicious side for almost any meal.

30-MINUTE
Serves: 2
Prep: 5 minutes
Cook: 25 minutes

Ingredients:
- 2 medium zucchini, halved lengthwise and seeded
- ¼ cup crushed pork rinds
- ¼ cup grated Parmesan cheese
- 2 garlic cloves, minced
- 2 tablespoons melted butter
- Pink salt
- Freshly ground black pepper
- Olive oil, for drizzling

Instructions:
1. Preheat the oven to 400°F. Line a baking sheet with aluminum foil or a silicone baking mat.

2. Place the zucchini halves, cut side up, on the prepared baking sheet.

3. In a medium bowl, combine crushed pork rinds, Parmesan cheese, minced garlic, and melted butter.

Season with pink salt and freshly ground black pepper, mixing until well blended.

4. Spoon the pork rind mixture evenly over each zucchini half, pressing lightly to adhere. Drizzle a little olive oil on top.

5. Bake for about 20 minutes, or until the topping is golden and crisp.

6. For extra browning, switch the oven to broil and cook for 3 to 5 minutes—watch closely to prevent burning. Serve immediately.

Ingredient Tip: If you want extra room for toppings, you can hollow out the zucchini halves slightly with a spoon before adding the pork rind mixture.

CHEESE CHIPS AND GUACAMOLE

Missing chips while on keto? These easy-to-make cheese chips are a fantastic substitute, and paired with fresh guacamole, they're even better than the real thing!

30-MINUTE • VEGETARIAN
Serves: 2
Prep: 10 minutes
Cook: 10 minutes

For the Cheese Chips:
- 1 cup shredded cheese (I use a Mexican blend)

For the Guacamole:
- 1 avocado, mashed

- Juice of ½ lime

- 1 teaspoon diced jalapeño

- 2 tablespoons chopped fresh cilantro leaves

- Pink salt

- Freshly ground black pepper

Instructions:
Cheese Chips:

1. Preheat the oven to 350°F. Line a baking sheet with parchment paper or a silicone baking mat.

2. Drop ¼-cup mounds of shredded cheese onto the baking sheet, spacing them well apart.

3. Bake until the edges turn brown and the centers are fully melted, about 7 minutes.

4. Transfer the pan to a cooling rack and allow the chips to crisp up for 5 minutes. (They will be floppy right out of the oven but will harden as they cool.)

Guacamole:

1. In a medium bowl, combine the mashed avocado, lime juice, diced jalapeño, and chopped cilantro. Season with pink salt and pepper, and mix well.

2. Serve the guacamole topped on the cheese chips.

Ingredient Tip: For an extra kick, add some diced jalapeños to the cheese before baking.

CAULIFLOWER "POTATO" SALAD

Cauliflower's versatility shines in this keto-friendly take on classic potato salad. While it won't fool anyone as a real potato salad, it's just as satisfying and delicious.

VEGETARIAN
Serves: 2
Prep: 10 minutes + 3 hours to chill
Cook: 25 minutes

Ingredients:
- ½ head cauliflower
- 1 tablespoon olive oil
- Pink salt
- Freshly ground black pepper
- ⅓ cup mayonnaise
- 1 tablespoon mustard
- ¼ cup diced dill pickles
- 1 teaspoon paprika

Instructions:
1. Preheat the oven to 400°F. Line a baking sheet with aluminum foil or a silicone baking mat.

2. Cut the cauliflower into 1-inch pieces (bite-sized pieces work best for that potato salad feel).

3. In a large bowl, toss the cauliflower with olive oil, pink salt, and freshly ground black pepper until evenly coated.

4. Spread the cauliflower pieces on the baking sheet in a single layer. Bake for 25 minutes, or until the cauliflower starts to brown, stirring or shaking the pan halfway through cooking to ensure even roasting.

5. Remove from the oven and let cool slightly. In a large bowl, mix the roasted cauliflower with mayonnaise, mustard, and diced dill pickles. Sprinkle paprika over the top.

6. Refrigerate for at least 3 hours before serving to allow the flavors to meld.

Variations:

- Top with chopped hardboiled eggs for extra richness.

- Stir in diced celery and minced white onion for additional crunch and flavor.

Ingredient Tip: Avoid using precut cauliflower florets, as the pieces might be uneven and affect the texture of the salad.

LOADED CAULIFLOWER MASHED "POTATOES"

Cauliflower is a keto staple, and in this recipe, it's transformed into creamy, loaded mashed "potatoes" that are just as comforting as the original.

30-MINUTE
Serves: 4
Prep: 10 minutes
Cook: 10 minutes

Ingredients:
- 1 head fresh cauliflower, cut into cubes

- 2 garlic cloves, minced

- 6 tablespoons butter

- 2 tablespoons sour cream

- Pink salt

- Freshly ground black pepper

- 1 cup shredded cheese (I use Colby Jack)

- 6 bacon slices, cooked and crumbled

Instructions:
1. Bring a large pot of water to a boil over high heat. Add the cauliflower cubes, reduce heat to medium-low, and simmer for 8 to 10 minutes, until fork-tender. (Alternatively, steam the cauliflower if you prefer.)

2. Drain the cauliflower in a colander, then spread it onto a paper towel-lined plate to absorb excess

moisture. Pat dry carefully—removing as much water as possible ensures your mash isn't runny.

3. Transfer the cauliflower to a food processor or blender. Add minced garlic, butter, and sour cream, then season with pink salt and freshly ground black pepper.

4. Blend for about 1 minute, stopping every 30 seconds to scrape down the sides for even mixing.

5. Divide the mash evenly into four small serving dishes. Top each serving with shredded cheese and crumbled bacon. The cheese should melt from the heat of the mash, but if you want, you can place the dishes under a broiler for 1 minute to warm and melt the cheese fully.

6. Serve warm and enjoy!

Variations:

- Swap the Colby Jack cheese for ¼ cup grated Parmesan. Top with chopped prosciutto and 3 tablespoons chopped chives. For crispy prosciutto, briefly broil before serving.

KETO BREAD

After experimenting with many keto-friendly bread recipes, I finally landed on this version. The texture is fantastic, and this basic loaf works perfectly as a foundation for both sweet and savory variations.

30-MINUTE • VEGETARIAN
Makes: 1 loaf (12 slices)
Prep: 5 minutes
Cook: 25 minutes

Ingredients:
- 5 tablespoons butter, at room temperature (divided)

- 6 large eggs, lightly beaten

- 1½ cups almond flour

- 3 teaspoons baking powder

- 1 scoop MCT oil powder (optional, flavorless and adds high-quality fats; I use Perfect Keto's MCT oil powder)

- Pinch of pink salt

Instructions:
1. Preheat your oven to 390°F. Grease a 9-by-5-inch loaf pan with 1 tablespoon of butter.

2. In a large bowl, combine the lightly beaten eggs, almond flour, remaining 4 tablespoons of butter, baking powder, MCT oil powder (if using), and a pinch of pink salt. Using a hand mixer, blend until the mixture is smooth and well incorporated.

3. Pour the batter into the prepared loaf pan, spreading it evenly.

4. Bake for 25 minutes, or until a toothpick inserted in the center comes out clean.

5. Allow the loaf to cool slightly before slicing. Serve as desired.

Variations:
- **Keto Pumpkin Bread:** Add ¼ can of pure pumpkin purée (be sure to use plain pumpkin, not pumpkin pie mix) to the batter. Mix in 2 to 3 teaspoons of liquid stevia for sweetness and 1 tablespoon of pumpkin pie spice (a blend of cinnamon, nutmeg, ginger, and allspice). Bake as directed.

- **Keto Chocolate Chip Bread:** Fold ½ cup keto-friendly chocolate chips (I prefer Lily's, sweetened with stevia) into the batter before baking.

Nutrition (Per Loaf):
Calories: 1973 | Total Fat: 178g | Carbs: 46g | Net Carbs: 27g | Fiber: 19g | Protein: 74g

Nutrition (Per Slice):
Calories: 165 | Total Fat: 15g | Carbs: 4g | Net Carbs: 2g | Fiber: 2g | Protein: 6g

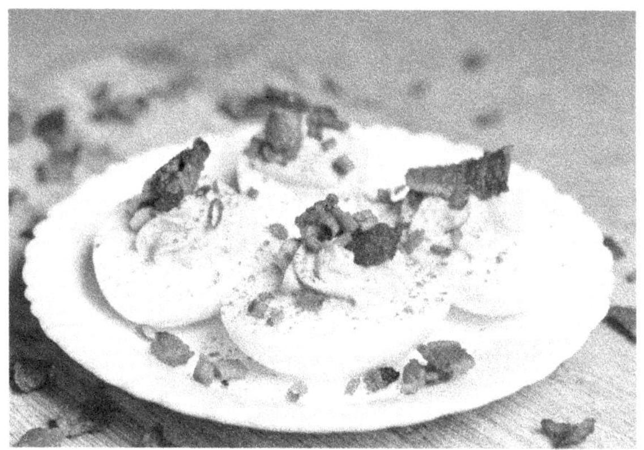

DEVILED EGGS

I have a long-standing love affair with deviled eggs. This particular recipe, which includes sour cream in the filling, elevates the classic into something truly special.

VEGETARIAN
Makes: 24 deviled egg halves
Prep: 30 minutes
Cook: 15 minutes

Ingredients:
- 12 large eggs

- ½ cup mayonnaise

- ¼ cup sour cream

- 1 tablespoon ground mustard

- Pink salt

- Freshly ground black pepper

- 1 teaspoon paprika

Instructions:

1. Place the eggs in a large saucepan and cover with 3 to 4 inches of water. Bring to a boil over high heat, then turn off the heat. Cover the pot and let the eggs sit for 15 minutes.

2. Drain the hot water and fill the pan with ice-cold water (adding ice cubes helps). Once cooled, gently tap each egg on the counter to crack the shell and peel under cold running water. Place peeled eggs on a paper towel-lined plate.

3. Slice each egg lengthwise and carefully scoop out the yolks into a small bowl. Mash the yolks until crumbly.

4. Add mayonnaise, sour cream, mustard, pink salt, and pepper to the yolks. Mix with a fork until smooth and creamy.

5. Spoon or pipe the yolk mixture back into the egg whites' hollowed centers. Sprinkle with paprika for color and serve.

Variations:
- **BLT Deviled Eggs:** Top each egg with crumbled bacon, chopped tomato, and chopped fresh basil (the "L" in BLT). These are crowd-pleasers for keto and non-keto eaters alike!

- **Bacon-Jalapeño Deviled Eggs:** Mix diced jalapeños (seeds removed for less heat) and crumbled bacon into the yolk filling.

- **Bacon-Avocado Deviled Eggs:** Add ½ avocado and 1 tablespoon fresh lime juice to the yolk mixture. Top with crumbled crispy bacon and swap paprika for Tajín seasoning (a flavorful blend of chile and lime).

Simplifying Tip:
To pipe the filling easily, use a zip-top sandwich bag and a drinking cup: place the bag in the cup with edges folded over, spoon in the filling, lift out, cut a small corner off the bag, and pipe away!

Nutrition (Per Batch):
Calories: 1775 | Total Fat: 159g | Carbs: 12g | Net Carbs: 11g | Fiber: 1g | Protein: 79g

Nutrition (Per Egg Half):
Calories: 74 | Total Fat: 7g | Carbs: 1g | Net Carbs: 0g | Fiber: 0g | Protein: 3g

CHICKEN-PECAN SALAD CUCUMBER BITES

Inspired by the classic Sonoma Chicken Salad at Whole Foods, this keto-friendly version removes grapes and adds fresh cucumber slices for a crunchy bite. Perfect for a light dinner or appetizer.

30-MINUTE • NO COOK
Serves: 2
Prep: 15 minutes

Ingredients:
- 1 cup cooked chicken breast, diced
- 2 tablespoons mayonnaise
- ¼ cup chopped pecans
- ¼ cup diced celery
- Pink salt
- Freshly ground black pepper
- 1 cucumber, peeled and sliced into ¼-inch rounds

Instructions:
1. In a medium bowl, combine diced chicken, mayonnaise, pecans, and celery. Season with pink salt and pepper, mixing well.

2. Arrange cucumber slices on a serving plate and sprinkle each with a pinch of pink salt.

3. Top each cucumber slice with a spoonful of the chicken-pecan salad mixture. Serve immediately or chilled.

Ingredient Tip:
These bites can be stored wrapped in the refrigerator for up to 2 days and will stay fresh and crunchy.

Nutrition (Per Batch):
Calories: 646 | Total Fat: 47g | Carbs: 12g | Net Carbs: 7g | Fiber: 5g | Protein: 46g

Nutrition (Per Serving):
Calories: 323 | Total Fat: 24g | Carbs: 6g | Net Carbs: 4g | Fiber: 3g | Protein: 23g

BUFFALO CHICKEN DIP

All the flavor of chicken wings packed into a creamy, spicy dip — perfect for game day or any gathering.

30-MINUTE
Serves: 2
Prep: 10 minutes
Cook: 20 minutes

Ingredients:
- Butter or olive oil, for greasing the pan
- 1 large cooked boneless chicken breast, shredded
- 8 ounces cream cheese
- ½ cup shredded Cheddar cheese
- ½ cup chunky blue cheese dressing
- ¼ cup buffalo wing sauce (I use Frank's RedHot Sauce)

Instructions:
1. Preheat the oven to 375°F. Grease a small baking dish.

2. In a medium bowl, mix shredded chicken, cream cheese, Cheddar cheese, blue cheese dressing, and buffalo wing sauce until well combined.

3. Transfer the mixture to the prepared baking dish, smoothing the top.

4. Bake for 20 minutes, until hot and bubbly.

5. Serve warm in a dip dish, perfect with celery sticks or pork rinds.

Nutrition (Per Batch):
Calories: 1717 | Total Fat: 145g | Carbs: 15g | Net Carbs: 15g | Fiber: 0g | Protein: 81g

Nutrition (Per Serving):
Calories: 859 | Total Fat: 73g | Carbs: 8g | Net Carbs: 8g | Fiber: 0g | Protein: 41g

ROASTED BRUSSELS SPROUTS WITH BACON

I didn't discover Brussels sprouts until my 30s, but roasted with bacon, they quickly became a favorite. This one-pan recipe is full of flavor and easy to prepare.

30-MINUTE
Serves: 2
Prep: 5 minutes
Cook: 25 minutes

Ingredients:

- ½ pound Brussels sprouts, cleaned, trimmed, and halved

- 1 tablespoon olive oil

- Pink salt

- Freshly ground black pepper

- 1 teaspoon red pepper flakes

- 6 bacon slices

- 1 tablespoon grated Parmesan cheese

Instructions:

1. Preheat oven to 400°F.

2. Toss Brussels sprouts in olive oil, pink salt, pepper, and red pepper flakes.

3. Cut bacon into 1-inch pieces using kitchen shears or a knife.

4. Spread Brussels sprouts and bacon pieces evenly on a baking sheet. Roast for about 25 minutes, stirring or shaking the pan halfway through for even cooking and crispiness.

5. Remove from oven, divide between two plates, and sprinkle with Parmesan cheese before serving.

Ingredient Tip:
Skip the Parmesan cheese to make this dish dairy-free.

Nutrition (Per Batch):
Calories: 496 | Total Fat: 36g | Carbs: 21g | Net Carbs: 13g | Fiber: 9g | Protein: 27g

Nutrition (Per Serving):
Calories: 248 | Total Fat: 18g | Carbs: 11g | Net Carbs: 7g | Fiber: 5g | Protein: 14g

SALAMI, PEPPERONCINI, AND CREAM CHEESE PINWHEELS

No cooking required for these flavorful, keto-friendly pinwheels—perfect for gatherings or quick snacks. Pepperoncini add a wonderful zing!

NO COOK
Serves: 2
Prep: 20 minutes + 6 hours chilling

Ingredients:
- 8 ounces cream cheese, at room temperature

- ¼ pound thinly sliced salami

- 2 tablespoons sliced pepperoncini (I use Mezzetta brand)

Instructions:
1. Lay a sheet of plastic wrap on a clean surface or cutting board.

2. Place the cream cheese in the center of the plastic wrap, then cover with another sheet of plastic wrap. Using a rolling pin, roll the cream cheese out evenly to about ¼-inch thickness, shaping roughly into a rectangle.

3. Remove the top layer of plastic wrap.

4. Arrange salami slices overlapping to cover the cream cheese completely.

5. Cover the salami with a fresh piece of plastic wrap, then carefully flip the entire layered rectangle so the

cream cheese side is now facing up. Remove the plastic wrap.

6. Spread sliced pepperoncini evenly over the cream cheese layer.

7. Roll the entire layered assembly tightly into a log, pressing gently to keep everything together. Wrap tightly in plastic wrap and refrigerate for at least 6 hours to set.

8. Slice into pinwheels and serve.

Ingredient Tip:
Feel free to swap the pepperoncini for chopped dill pickles, scallions, jalapeños, or sliced bell pepper for different flavor profiles.

Nutrition (Per Batch):
Calories: 1166 | Total Fat: 107g | Carbs: 13g | Net Carbs: 13g | Fiber: 0g | Protein: 38g

Nutrition (Per Serving):
Calories: 583 | Total Fat: 54g | Carbs: 7g | Net Carbs: 7g | Fiber: 0g | Protein: 19g

CAULIFLOWER STEAKS WITH BACON AND BLUE CHEESE

Inspired by the classic wedge salad, this warm, caramelized cauliflower steak topped with chunky blue cheese dressing and crispy bacon is a keto-friendly twist that's bursting with flavor.

30-MINUTE • ONE PAN • VEGETARIAN
Serves: 2
Prep: 5 minutes
Cook: 20 minutes

Ingredients:
- ½ head cauliflower

- 1 tablespoon olive oil

- Pink salt

- Freshly ground black pepper

- 4 bacon slices

- 2 tablespoons blue cheese salad dressing (I use Trader Joe's Chunky Blue Cheese Dressing)

Instructions:
1. Preheat oven to 425°F. Line a baking sheet with aluminum foil or a silicone baking mat.

2. Remove and discard the cauliflower leaves, then cut into 1-inch-thick slices (steaks). Reserve any loose florets to roast alongside.

3. Place cauliflower steaks and florets on the baking sheet. Lightly brush the cauliflower with olive oil,

season with pink salt and pepper. Arrange bacon
slices on the same pan.

4. Roast everything for 20 minutes, until cauliflower is
    caramelized and bacon is crispy.

5. Plate the cauliflower steaks, drizzle with blue
    cheese dressing, sprinkle with crumbled bacon, and
    serve immediately.

Substitution Tip:
You can use cabbage steaks instead of cauliflower for a
similar preparation.

Nutrition (Per Batch):
Calories: 507 | Total Fat: 38g | Carbs: 22g | Net Carbs: 14g |
Fiber: 8g | Protein: 22g

Nutrition (Per Serving):
Calories: 254 | Total Fat: 19g | Carbs: 11g | Net Carbs: 7g |
Fiber: 4g | Protein: 11g

BACON-WRAPPED JALAPEÑOS

Perfect game day snack when I'm glued to watching the Denver Broncos in the fall and winter. Simple ingredients, great flavor—but prep takes some time. (I get my daughter to help prep so I don't miss the game!)

30-MINUTE • ONE PAN
Serves: 4
Prep: 10 minutes
Cook: 20 minutes

Ingredients:
- 10 jalapeños

- 8 ounces cream cheese, room temperature

- 1 pound bacon (approximately half a slice per popper)

Instructions:
1. Preheat oven to 450°F. Line a baking sheet with aluminum foil or a silicone baking mat.

2. Halve the jalapeños lengthwise and remove seeds and membranes for less heat (leave them in if you prefer extra spice). Arrange jalapeño halves cut-side up on the baking sheet.

3. Fill each jalapeño half with cream cheese.

4. Wrap each stuffed jalapeño half with a slice (or half slice, depending on size) of bacon. Secure with 1 to 2 toothpicks to hold the bacon in place while baking.

5. Bake for 20 minutes or until bacon is crispy and cooked through.

6. Serve warm or at room temperature—both are delicious!

Ingredient Tip:
Wear thin rubber gloves when prepping jalapeños to avoid irritation from the chile pepper oils. Wash hands thoroughly and avoid touching your face or eyes.

Nutrition (Per Batch):
Calories: 3272 | Total Fat: 268g | Carbs: 24g | Net Carbs: 20g | Fiber: 4g | Protein: 183g

Nutrition (Per Serving):
Calories: 164 | Total Fat: 13g | Carbs: 1g | Net Carbs: 1g | Fiber: 0g | Protein: 9g

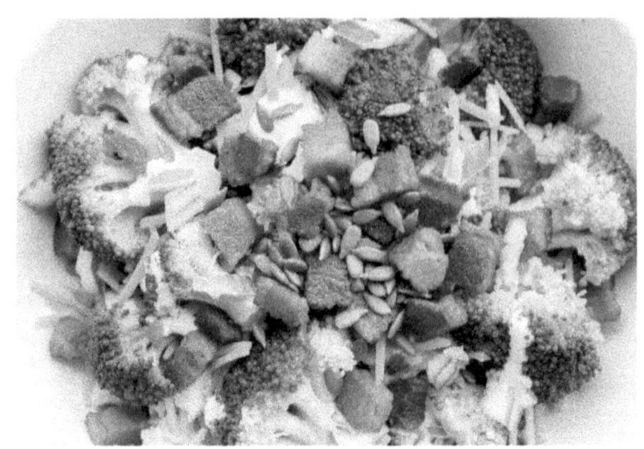

CREAMY BROCCOLI-BACON SALAD

This fresh, creamy, and crunchy cold salad is a perfect side dish for grilled meats, fish, or any light, summer-friendly entrée. The raw broccoli provides a satisfying crunch, while the honey mustard dressing adds a subtle sweet kick that balances the salty flavors beautifully.

Serves: 2
Prep: 10 minutes, plus at least 1 hour chilling
Cook: 10 minutes

Ingredients:
- 6 bacon slices

- ½ pound fresh broccoli, cut into small florets

- ½ cup sliced almonds

- ⅓ cup mayonnaise

- 1 tablespoon honey mustard dressing

Instructions:
1. Heat a large skillet over medium-high heat. Add the bacon slices and cook them on both sides until crispy, about 8 minutes total.

2. Once cooked, transfer the bacon to a paper towel–lined plate to drain excess fat and cool for about 5 minutes. When cool enough to handle, crumble the bacon into bite-sized pieces.

3. In a large mixing bowl, combine the fresh broccoli florets, sliced almonds, and bacon crumbles.

4. In a small bowl, whisk together the mayonnaise and honey mustard dressing until smooth and well blended.

CHAPTER 5
FISH & POULTRY ENTRÉES

Chicken and fish are staples in my kitchen. They're incredibly versatile, easy to work with, and perfect for adding healthy fats and bold flavors that fit beautifully into a ketogenic lifestyle. In this chapter, you'll find a variety of dishes—some crunchy, some creamy, some light, and others rich and indulgent.

Each entrée is satisfying on its own, but they also pair wonderfully with the sides from Chapter 4. Whether you're cooking a quick weeknight dinner or something special you will want to make again and again, these recipes are designed to be simple, flavorful, and keto-approved.

Baked Lemon-Butter Fish
Fish Taco Bowl
Scallops with Creamy Bacon Sauce
Shrimp and Avocado Lettuce Cups
Garlic Butter Shrimp
Parmesan-Garlic Salmon with Asparagus
Seared-Salmon Shirataki Rice Bowls
Pork Rind Salmon Cakes
Creamy Dill Salmon
Chicken-Basil Alfredo with Shirataki Noodles
Chicken Quesadilla
Garlic-Parmesan Chicken Wings
Chicken Skewers with Peanut Sauce
Braised Chicken Thighs with Kalamata Olives
Buttery Garlic Chicken
Cheesy Bacon and Broccoli Chicken
Parmesan Baked Chicken

Crunchy Chicken Milanese
Baked Garlic and Paprika Chicken Legs
Creamy Slow-Cooker Chicken

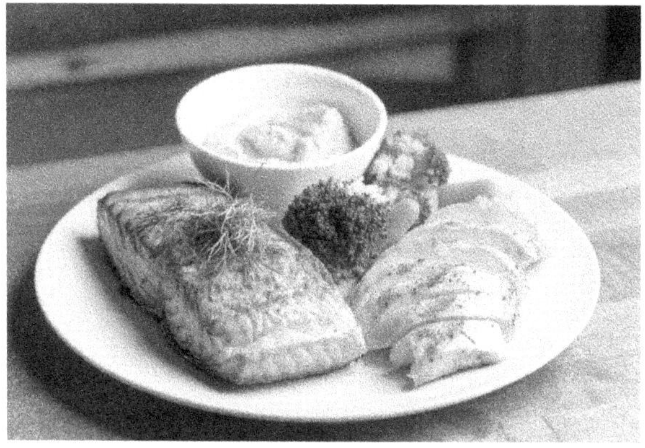

BAKED LEMON-BUTTER FISH

Buttery, flaky fish is something I could eat any day of the week. The lemon brightens up the mild flavor of the fish, while the capers add a salty, zesty pop that ties everything together.

30-Minute • Serves 2
Prep: 10 minutes
Cook: 20 minutes

Ingredients

- 4 tablespoons butter, plus more for greasing
- 2 (5-ounce) tilapia fillets
- Pink salt
- Freshly ground black pepper
- 2 garlic cloves, minced
- 1 lemon, zested and juiced
- 2 tablespoons capers, rinsed and chopped

Instructions

1. Preheat the oven to 400°F. Lightly coat an 8-inch baking dish with butter.
2. Pat the tilapia fillets dry with paper towels. Season both sides evenly with pink salt and black pepper, then place them in the prepared baking dish.
3. In a medium skillet over medium heat, melt the butter. Add the minced garlic and cook for 3 to 5 minutes, stirring frequently, until fragrant and lightly golden (do not let it burn).
4. Remove the skillet from the heat and stir in the lemon zest and 2 tablespoons of lemon juice.

5. Pour the lemon-butter sauce evenly over the fish and sprinkle the chopped capers around the dish.
6. Bake for 12 to 15 minutes, until the fish flakes easily with a fork. Serve immediately.

Substitution Tip: This recipe works well with any mild white fish. Salmon is also delicious with the lemon-butter sauce.

FISH TACO BOWL

This Fish Taco Bowl packs bold flavor into just a few ingredients. Tajín seasoning adds chile, lime, and salt in one step, while crunchy cabbage and creamy avocado create the perfect contrast.

30-Minute • Serves 2
Prep: 10 minutes
Cook: 15 minutes

Ingredients

- 2 (5-ounce) tilapia fillets
- 1 tablespoon olive oil
- 4 teaspoons Tajín seasoning salt, divided
- 2 cups presliced coleslaw cabbage mix
- 1 tablespoon Spicy Red Pepper Miso Mayo, plus more for serving
- 1 avocado, mashed
- Pink salt
- Freshly ground black pepper

Instructions

1. Preheat the oven to 425°F. Line a baking sheet with aluminum foil or a silicone baking mat.

2. Rub the tilapia fillets with olive oil, then coat evenly with 2 teaspoons of Tajín seasoning. Place the fish on the prepared baking sheet.
3. Bake for about 15 minutes, until the fish is opaque and flakes easily. Transfer to a cooling rack and let rest for 4 minutes.
4. In a medium bowl, gently toss the coleslaw mix with the mayo—just enough to lightly coat the cabbage.
5. Add the mashed avocado and remaining 2 teaspoons of Tajín. Season with pink salt and pepper, then divide the slaw between two bowls.
6. Use two forks to flake the fish into bite-sized pieces and add it to the bowls.
7. Finish with a drizzle of extra mayo sauce and serve.

Ingredient Tip: Avocado-Lime Crema works well if you don't have Spicy Red Pepper Miso Mayo.

SCALLOPS WITH CREAMY BACON SAUCE

Large sea scallops cooked just right and topped with a rich bacon cream sauce make this dish feel luxurious while staying keto-friendly.

30-Minute • Serves 2
Prep: 5 minutes
Cook: 20 minutes

Instructions (condensed for readability, fully detailed retained)

1. Cook bacon in a skillet until crisp; transfer to paper towels.
2. Reduce heat, then add cream, butter, and Parmesan to the bacon fat. Stir constantly until thickened and reduced by half.
3. Heat ghee in a separate skillet. Season scallops and sear for 1 minute per side until golden.
4. Plate cream sauce, crumble bacon on top, add scallops, and serve immediately.

Variation Tip: A squeeze of lemon juice or a handful of wilted spinach adds freshness to the richness.

SHRIMP AND AVOCADO LETTUCE CUPS

These lettuce cups are light, refreshing, and fun to eat—perfect for a quick lunch or easy dinner.

30-Minute • One Pan • Serves 2

Instructions

1. Heat ghee in a skillet and warm shrimp just until heated through. Season lightly.
2. Season tomatoes and avocado separately.
3. Fill lettuce leaves with shrimp, tomatoes, and avocado. Drizzle with mayo and serve.

GARLIC BUTTER SHRIMP

This one-pan dish delivers big flavor fast—juicy shrimp swimming in garlic butter and bright lemon.

30-Minute • One Pan • Serves 2

Instructions

1. Melt butter in a baking dish while the oven preheats.
2. Add shrimp, garlic, lemon slices, and seasoning.
3. Bake, stirring halfway, then finish with fresh lemon juice.

PARMESAN-GARLIC SALMON WITH ASPARAGUS

This is one of my go-to weeknight meals—simple, filling, and packed with flavor.

30-Minute • One Pan • Serves 2

Instructions

1. Season salmon and arrange on a lined baking sheet with asparagus.
2. Prepare garlic butter and drizzle over everything.
3. Sprinkle Parmesan on top.
4. Bake until salmon is cooked through and asparagus is tender-crisp. Broil briefly if desired.

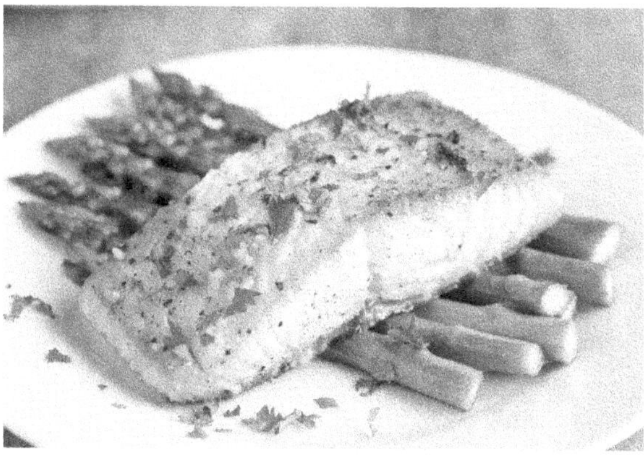

SEARED SALMON SHIRATAKI RICE BOWLS

I love poke bowls. I eat them often because raw salmon is one of my favorite foods. While this dish can't technically be called "poke," it is inspired by the same fresh, savory flavors—soy sauce, creamy avocado, crisp cucumber, and tender salmon—served over low-carb shirataki rice.

SERVES 2
PREP: 10 minutes, plus 30 minutes to marinate
COOK: 10 minutes

Ingredients
- 2 (6-ounce) salmon fillets, skin on

- 4 tablespoons soy sauce or coconut aminos, divided

- 2 small Persian cucumbers or ½ large English cucumber

- 1 tablespoon ghee

- 1 (8-ounce) package Miracle Shirataki Rice

- 1 avocado, diced

- Pink salt

- Freshly ground black pepper

Instructions
1. Place the salmon fillets in an 8-inch baking dish. Pour 3 tablespoons of the soy sauce over the salmon, turning gently to coat. Cover the dish and marinate in the refrigerator for 30 minutes.

2. While the salmon marinates, thinly slice the cucumbers and place them in a small bowl. Add the remaining 1 tablespoon of soy sauce, toss to combine, and set aside.

3. Heat a medium skillet over medium heat and melt the ghee. Add the salmon fillets skin-side down. Spoon a small amount of the marinade over the fish, then sear for 3 to 4 minutes per side, until the salmon is lightly browned on the outside and just cooked through. Remove from heat.

4. Meanwhile, prepare the shirataki rice according to the package instructions:

   o Rinse the rice thoroughly under cold water using a colander.

   o Bring a saucepan of water to a boil. Add the rice and boil for 2 minutes.

   o Drain the rice well and return the empty saucepan to the stove.

   o Add the drained rice to the dry pan and dry-roast over medium heat, stirring frequently, until all excess moisture evaporates and the rice looks dry and opaque.

5. Season the diced avocado lightly with pink salt and pepper.

6. Place the cooked salmon on a plate and carefully remove the skin. Cut the salmon into bite-size pieces.

7. To assemble the bowls, divide the shirataki rice between two bowls. Top each bowl with marinated cucumbers, avocado, and salmon. Serve immediately.

Variations

One of the best parts of a poke-style bowl is customizing the toppings. Try adding:

- Miso mayo

- Furikake (sesame seed and seaweed seasoning)

- Fresh cooked crab

- Sliced scallions

- Thinly sliced fresh ginger

- Wasabi

PORK RIND SALMON CAKES

This easy fish-cake recipe uses canned salmon, making it quick and convenient. I love using Wild Planet's canned salmon because it's fresh-caught wild pink salmon with excellent flavor. Crushed pork rinds replace breadcrumbs, adding structure and extra flavor while keeping the recipe keto-friendly.

30-MINUTE
SERVES 2
PREP: 10 minutes
COOK: 10 minutes

Ingredients

- 6 ounces canned Alaska wild salmon, drained

- 2 tablespoons crushed pork rinds

- 1 egg, lightly beaten

- 3 tablespoons mayonnaise, divided

- Pink salt

- Freshly ground black pepper

- 1 tablespoon ghee

- ½ tablespoon Dijon mustard

Instructions

1. In a medium bowl, combine the salmon, crushed pork rinds, egg, and 1½ tablespoons of the mayonnaise. Season with pink salt and pepper and mix until well combined.

2. Using your hands, shape the mixture into small patties, about the size of hockey pucks or slightly smaller. Press firmly so the patties hold together.

3. Heat a medium skillet over medium-high heat and melt the ghee. Once sizzling, add the salmon patties. Cook for about 3 minutes per side, until golden brown and heated through.

4. Transfer the cooked patties to a paper towel–lined plate to absorb excess grease.

5. In a small bowl, mix the remaining 1½ tablespoons of mayonnaise with the Dijon mustard.

6. Serve the salmon cakes warm with the mayo-mustard dipping sauce on the side.

Ingredient Tip: Choose wild-caught salmon whenever possible. Salmon labeled "Atlantic" is typically farmed, so always check the label.

CREAMY DILL SALMON

Salmon is my favorite food in all its forms—smoked, baked, or seared. This creamy dill salmon is incredibly easy to prepare and perfect for entertaining. Using mayonnaise keeps the fish juicy while adding rich flavor, and fresh dill gives it a bright, herbal finish.

30-MINUTE
ONE PAN
SERVES 2
PREP: 10 minutes
COOK: 10 minutes

Ingredients

- 2 tablespoons ghee, melted

- 2 (6-ounce) salmon fillets, skin on

- Pink salt

- Freshly ground black pepper

- ¼ cup mayonnaise

- 1 tablespoon Dijon mustard

- 2 tablespoons minced fresh dill

- Pinch garlic powder

Instructions

1. Preheat the oven to 450°F. Coat a 9-by-13-inch baking dish evenly with the melted ghee.

2. Pat the salmon fillets dry with paper towels. Season both sides with pink salt and pepper, then place them skin-side down in the prepared dish.

3. In a small bowl, stir together the mayonnaise, Dijon mustard, dill, and garlic powder.

4. Spread the mayonnaise mixture evenly over the tops of the salmon fillets, fully coating the surface.

5. Bake for 7 to 9 minutes, depending on your preference—7 minutes for medium-rare or 9 minutes for well-done. Serve immediately.

Ingredient Tip: Salmon skin contains a high concentration of healthy fats and helps keep the fish moist during cooking.

CHICKEN-BASIL ALFREDO WITH SHIRATAKI NOODLES

Shirataki noodles can be puzzling at first, but once you understand the process, they become a fantastic low-carb pasta alternative. This rich, comforting dish combines creamy Alfredo sauce, tender chicken, and fresh basil for a deeply satisfying keto meal.

30-MINUTE
SERVES 2
PREP: 10 minutes
COOK: 15 minutes

Ingredients
For the Noodles

- 1 (7-ounce) package Miracle Noodle Fettuccini Shirataki Noodles

For the Sauce

- 1 tablespoon olive oil

- 4 ounces cooked shredded chicken (rotisserie works well)

- Pink salt

- Freshly ground black pepper

- 1 cup Alfredo sauce

- ¼ cup grated Parmesan cheese

- 2 tablespoons chopped fresh basil

Instructions

Prepare the Noodles

1. Rinse the noodles thoroughly under cold water in a colander to remove their natural odor.

2. Bring a large saucepan of water to a boil. Add the noodles and boil for 2 minutes, then drain.

3. Transfer the drained noodles to a large, dry skillet over medium-low heat. Do not add oil. Cook, stirring frequently, until all moisture evaporates. Remove from heat and set aside.

Prepare the Sauce

4. In the same saucepan, heat the olive oil over medium heat. Add the shredded chicken and season with pink salt and pepper.

5. Pour the Alfredo sauce over the chicken and cook until warmed through. Adjust seasoning as needed.

6. Add the dried noodles to the sauce and toss until evenly coated.

7. Divide between two plates, top with Parmesan cheese and fresh basil, and serve.

Substitution Tip: For a vegetarian version, replace the chicken with sautéed mushrooms.

CHICKEN QUESADILLA

There's something endlessly comforting about a chicken quesadilla. Thanks to low-carb tortillas, this classic favorite fits beautifully into a keto lifestyle.

30-MINUTE
ONE PAN
SERVES 2
PREP: 5 minutes
COOK: 5 minutes

Ingredients

- 1 tablespoon olive oil

- 2 low-carbohydrate tortillas

- ½ cup shredded Mexican-blend cheese

- 2 ounces shredded chicken

- 1 teaspoon Tajín seasoning salt

- 2 tablespoons sour cream

Instructions

1. Heat the olive oil in a large skillet over medium-high heat. Place one tortilla in the pan.

2. Layer the tortilla with half the cheese, the chicken, the Tajín seasoning, and the remaining cheese. Top with the second tortilla.

3. Cook for about 2 minutes, checking underneath until the bottom tortilla is golden and the cheese begins to melt. Flip carefully and cook the second side for about 1 minute.

4. Transfer the quesadilla to a cutting board and let
    rest for 2 minutes before slicing into wedges.

5. Serve half the quesadilla per plate with sour cream.

GARLIC-PARMESAN CHICKEN WINGS

These slow-cooker chicken wings are rich, buttery, and
incredibly aromatic. Finishing them under the broiler gives
them that irresistible crispy finish.

SERVES 2
PREP: 10 minutes
COOK: 3 hours

Ingredients
- 8 tablespoons (1 stick) butter

- 2 garlic cloves, minced

- 1 tablespoon dried Italian seasoning

- ¼ cup grated Parmesan cheese, plus ½ cup more

- Pink salt

- Freshly ground black pepper

- 1 pound chicken wings

Instructions
1. Place the slow-cooker insert into the base and set to
    high. Line a baking sheet with foil or a silicone mat.

2. Add the butter, garlic, Italian seasoning, and ¼ cup
    Parmesan cheese to the slow cooker. Season with
    pink salt and pepper. Allow the butter to melt, then
    stir to combine.

3. Add the chicken wings and toss until fully coated in the butter mixture.

4. Cover and cook for 2 hours and 45 minutes.

5. Preheat the broiler.

6. Transfer the wings to the prepared baking sheet. Sprinkle with the remaining ½ cup Parmesan cheese.

7. Broil for about 5 minutes, until the wings are crispy and golden. Serve hot.

CHICKEN SKEWERS WITH PEANUT SAUCE

A traditional chicken satay usually contains many more ingredients, so I'm not calling this dish a true satay—though it is clearly inspired by those classic flavors. I don't eat peanut butter often, but when it's paired with spice and sesame, it becomes irresistible. Adjust the Sriracha to control the heat level to your liking.

SERVES 2
PREP: 10 minutes, plus 1 hour to marinate
COOK: 15 minutes

Ingredients

- 1 pound boneless, skinless chicken breast, cut into bite-size chunks

- 3 tablespoons soy sauce or coconut aminos, divided

- ½ teaspoon Sriracha sauce, plus ¼ teaspoon

- 3 teaspoons toasted sesame oil, divided

- Ghee, for greasing

- 2 tablespoons peanut butter

- Pink salt

- Freshly ground black pepper

Instructions

1. Place the chicken chunks in a large zip-top bag. Add 2 tablespoons of the soy sauce, ½ teaspoon of the Sriracha, and 2 teaspoons of the sesame oil. Seal the bag and massage gently to coat the chicken

evenly. Refrigerate and marinate for at least 1 hour or up to overnight.

2. If using wooden skewers, soak them in water for 30 minutes to prevent burning.

3. Preheat a grill pan, outdoor grill, or large skillet over low heat. Lightly grease the surface with ghee.

4. Thread the marinated chicken chunks evenly onto the skewers.

5. Place the skewers on the grill or skillet and cook for 10 to 15 minutes, turning halfway through, until the chicken is fully cooked and lightly charred.

6. While the chicken cooks, prepare the peanut sauce. In a small bowl, whisk together the remaining 1 tablespoon soy sauce, ¼ teaspoon Sriracha, 1 teaspoon sesame oil, and peanut butter. Season lightly with pink salt and pepper.

7. Serve the chicken skewers hot with the peanut sauce on the side for dipping.

Ingredient Tip: Coconut aminos taste similar to soy sauce but are gluten-free and Paleo-friendly.

BRAISED CHICKEN THIGHS WITH KALAMATA OLIVES

Chicken thighs are incredibly flavorful and forgiving, but they do require a bit of technique. The secret is starting them skin-side down on the stovetop to develop crispy skin before finishing them in the oven. A cast-iron skillet or other oven-safe pan works best.

ONE PAN
SERVES 2
PREP: 10 minutes
COOK: 40 minutes

Ingredients

- 4 chicken thighs, skin on

- Pink salt

- Freshly ground black pepper

- 2 tablespoons ghee

- ½ cup chicken broth

- 1 lemon, half sliced and half juiced

- ½ cup pitted Kalamata olives

- 2 tablespoons butter

Instructions

1. Preheat the oven to 375°F.

2. Pat the chicken thighs dry with paper towels and season generously with pink salt and pepper.

3. Heat the ghee in an oven-safe skillet over medium-high heat. Once hot, place the chicken thighs skin-side down and cook undisturbed for about 8 minutes, until the skin is deeply golden and crispy.

4. Flip the chicken thighs and cook for 2 minutes on the second side.

5. Carefully pour the chicken broth around the thighs. Add the lemon slices, lemon juice, and olives to the pan.

6. Transfer the skillet to the oven and bake for about 30 minutes, until the chicken is fully cooked and tender.

7. Stir the butter into the pan juices just before serving.

8. Divide the chicken and olives between two plates and spoon the pan sauce over the top.

Ingredient Tip: Feel free to substitute your favorite olives if Kalamata olives aren't available.

BUTTERY GARLIC CHICKEN

Chicken drenched in butter? Absolutely. This dish is rich, moist, and deeply satisfying. Be sure to spoon the garlic butter over the chicken before serving—it's too good to waste.

SERVES 2
PREP: 5 minutes
COOK: 40 minutes

Ingredients
- 2 tablespoons ghee, melted

- 2 boneless, skinless chicken breasts

- Pink salt

- Freshly ground black pepper

- 1 tablespoon dried Italian seasoning

- 4 tablespoons butter

- 2 garlic cloves, minced

- ¼ cup grated Parmesan cheese

Instructions
1. Preheat the oven to 375°F. Lightly coat a baking dish large enough to hold both chicken breasts with the melted ghee.

2. Pat the chicken breasts dry and season both sides with pink salt, pepper, and Italian seasoning. Place them in the baking dish.

3. In a medium skillet over medium heat, melt the butter. Add the minced garlic and cook for about 5 minutes, stirring frequently, until lightly golden but not burned.

4. Pour the garlic-butter mixture evenly over the chicken.

5. Bake for 30 to 35 minutes, until the chicken is cooked through.

6. Sprinkle Parmesan cheese over the chicken and let it rest in the baking dish for 5 minutes.

7. Serve with the butter sauce spooned generously over the top.

CHEESY BACON AND BROCCOLI CHICKEN

Anything topped with cream cheese and bacon is bound to be delicious. While this recipe includes steps for cooking everything from scratch, it's also perfect for using leftover chicken and bacon.

SERVES 2
PREP: 10 minutes
COOK: 1 hour

Instructions

1. Preheat the oven to 375°F.

2. Grease a baking dish with ghee.

3. Pat the chicken breasts dry and season with pink salt and pepper.

4. Place the chicken and bacon in the dish and bake for 25 minutes.

5. Remove the chicken and shred it using two forks. Season again lightly.

6. Transfer the bacon to a paper towel–lined plate and crumble once crisp.

7. In a bowl, mix the shredded chicken, cream cheese, broccoli, and half the bacon.

8. Transfer the mixture back to the baking dish. Top with Cheddar cheese and remaining bacon.

9. Bake for about 35 minutes, until the cheese is bubbling and lightly browned.

PARMESAN BAKED CHICKEN

This is one of the simplest and most reliable chicken recipes I know. Mayonnaise keeps the chicken juicy, while pork rinds add a crunchy, keto-friendly topping.

30-MINUTE | ONE PAN | SERVES 2

Instructions

1. Preheat the oven to 425°F and grease a baking dish with ghee.

2. Season the chicken breasts with pink salt and pepper and place in the dish.

3. Mix the mayonnaise, Parmesan, and Italian seasoning.

4. Spread evenly over the chicken and top with crushed pork rinds.

5. Bake for about 20 minutes, until golden and cooked through.

CRUNCHY CHICKEN MILANESE

This crispy chicken is always a crowd-pleaser. Pounding the chicken thin ensures quick cooking and maximum crunch.

30-MINUTE | SERVES 2

Instructions

1. Pound the chicken breasts to about ½ inch thickness.

2. Prepare a breading station with seasoned coconut flour, beaten egg, and crushed pork rinds.

3. Coat each chicken breast in flour, then egg, then pork rinds.

4. Cook in hot olive oil for 3 to 5 minutes per side until golden and cooked through.

BAKED GARLIC AND PAPRIKA CHICKEN LEGS

Crispy chicken drumsticks layered with garlic, paprika, and herbs make this dish worth every minute of roasting.

SERVES 2

Instructions

1. Preheat oven to 425°F and line a baking pan.

2. Season chicken thoroughly with salt and pepper.

3. Warm ghee with garlic, paprika, and herbs.

4. Coat chicken, bake, add green beans halfway, and roast until crispy.

CREAMY SLOW-COOKER CHICKEN

This comforting slow-cooker meal fills the kitchen with rich aromas while cooking gently to tender perfection.

SERVES 2

Instructions
1. Brown chicken in ghee.

2. Transfer to slow cooker and set to low.

3. Mix sauce ingredients and pour over chicken.

4. Cook for 4 hours, then add spinach and cook 5 minutes more.

CHAPTER SIX
PORK & BEEF ENTRÉES

When most people think of the ketogenic lifestyle, pork and beef are often the first foods that come to mind—and for good reason. These proteins are naturally low in carbohydrates, deeply satisfying, and incredibly versatile. This chapter features a range of flavorful pork and beef dishes designed to fit effortlessly into busy schedules.

From slow-cooker meals you can set and forget to quick, weeknight-friendly recipes ready in under 30 minutes, these entrées prove that keto cooking can be both simple and delicious. Each dish delivers bold flavor with minimal ingredients, making it easy to enjoy hearty, comforting meals without spending hours in the kitchen.

Recipes in this chapter include:
BLTA Cups
Butter and Herb Pork Chops
 Parmesan Pork Chops and Roasted Asparagus
Sesame Pork and Green Beans
Slow-Cooker Barbecue Ribs
 Kalua Pork with Cabbage
 Pork Burgers with Sriracha Mayo
 Blue Cheese Pork Chops
Carnitas
Carnitas Nachos
Pepperoni Low-Carb Tortilla Pizza
Beef and Broccoli Roast
 Beef and Bell Pepper "Potato Skins"
Skirt Steak with Chimichurri Sauce
 Barbacoa Beef Roast
Steak and Egg Bibimbap
 Mississippi Pot Roast

Taco Cheese Cups
 Bacon Cheeseburger Casserole
Feta-Stuffed Burgers

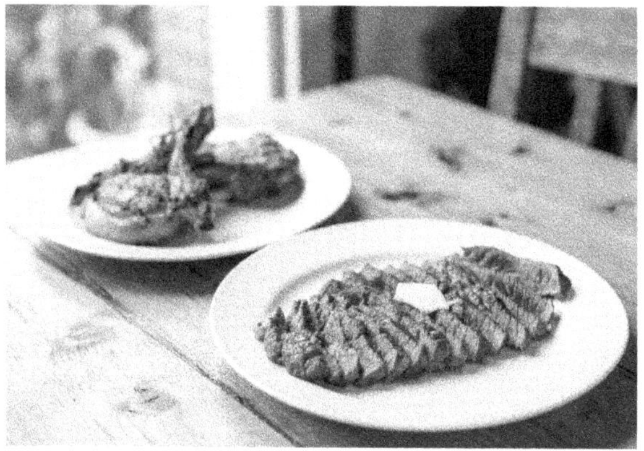

BLTA CUPS

What's better than a cup made entirely of bacon? In my opinion, very little. Bacon pairs beautifully with almost anything, but the classic combination of bacon, lettuce, tomato, and avocado never disappoints. These crispy bacon cups are packed with flavor and make a fun, satisfying meal or appetizer.

ONE PAN
Serves: 2
Prep: 5 minutes
Cook: 20 minutes, plus 10 minutes to rest

Ingredients:

- 12 bacon slices

- ¼ head romaine lettuce, chopped

- ½ avocado, diced

- ½ cup grape tomatoes, halved

- 2 tablespoons sour cream

Instructions:

1. Preheat the oven to 400°F. You will need a muffin tin. A jumbo muffin tin works best, but a standard muffin tin will also work.

2. Turn the muffin tin upside down and place it on a baking sheet. Create a cross using two halved bacon strips over one muffin cup. Add two more bacon halves around the perimeter. Wrap one full bacon strip around the base of the muffin cup and secure it tightly with a toothpick.

3. Repeat the process to form a total of four bacon cups.

4. Bake for 20 minutes, or until the bacon is deeply golden and crisp.

5. Carefully transfer the bacon cups to a cooling rack and let them rest for at least 10 minutes to firm up.

6. Once set, gently remove the bacon cups from the muffin tin. Place two cups on each plate.

7. Fill each cup with chopped romaine, then top with avocado, tomatoes, and a dollop of sour cream. Serve immediately.

INGREDIENT TIP: The bacon cups can be made ahead and stored, covered, in the refrigerator for up to 3 days.

Per Batch:
Calories: 708; Total Fat: 56g; Carbs: 13g; Net Carbs: 6g; Fiber: 7g; Protein: 39g

Per Serving:
Calories: 354; Total Fat: 28g; Carbs: 6.5g; Net Carbs: 3g; Fiber: 3.5g; Protein: 19.5g

BUTTER AND HERB PORK CHOPS

Sometimes the simplest flavors truly shine the brightest. Butter, herbs, and olive oil come together effortlessly in this dish to highlight the natural richness of pork. These pork chops bake quickly, making them perfect for an easy yet elegant weeknight dinner.

30-MINUTE • ONE PAN
Serves: 2
Prep: 5 minutes
Cook: 25 minutes

Ingredients:

- 1 tablespoon butter, plus more for greasing

- 2 boneless pork chops

- Pink salt

- Freshly ground black pepper

- 1 tablespoon dried Italian seasoning

- 1 tablespoon chopped fresh flat-leaf parsley

- 1 tablespoon olive oil

Instructions:

1. Preheat the oven to 350°F. Lightly coat a baking dish large enough to hold both pork chops with butter.

2. Pat the pork chops dry with a paper towel and place them in the prepared baking dish. Season both sides

generously with pink salt, pepper, and Italian seasoning.

3. Sprinkle the fresh parsley evenly over the pork chops. Drizzle the olive oil over each chop, then place ½ tablespoon of butter on top of each one.

4. Bake for 20 to 25 minutes, depending on thickness, until the pork is fully cooked and tender.

5. Transfer the pork chops to two plates. Spoon the buttery pan juices over the top and serve hot.

SERVING TIP: These pork chops pair especially well with mashed cauliflower.

Per Batch:
Calories: 666; Total Fat: 45g; Carbs: 0g; Net Carbs: 0g; Fiber: 0g; Protein: 62g

Per Serving:
Calories: 333; Total Fat: 23g; Carbs: 0g; Net Carbs: 0g; Fiber: 0g; Protein: 31g

PARMESAN PORK CHOPS AND ROASTED ASPARAGUS

This one-pan dinner is ideal for busy evenings when you want something satisfying with minimal cleanup. The pork chops are coated in a crispy Parmesan and pork rind crust, while the asparagus roasts alongside them for a perfectly balanced meal.

ONE PAN
Serves: 2
Prep: 10 minutes
Cook: 25 minutes

Ingredients:

- ¼ cup grated Parmesan cheese

- ¼ cup crushed pork rinds

- 1 teaspoon garlic powder

- 2 boneless pork chops

- Pink salt

- Freshly ground black pepper

- Olive oil, for drizzling

- ½ pound asparagus spears, tough ends removed

Instructions:

1. Preheat the oven to 350°F. Line a baking sheet with aluminum foil or a silicone baking mat.

2. In a medium bowl, combine the Parmesan cheese, crushed pork rinds, and garlic powder.

3. Pat the pork chops dry with a paper towel and season both sides with pink salt and pepper.

4. Press each pork chop firmly into the Parmesan mixture, coating both sides well. Place the coated pork chops on the prepared baking sheet.

5. Drizzle a small amount of olive oil over each pork chop.

6. Arrange the asparagus around the pork chops on the baking sheet. Drizzle with olive oil and season with pink salt and pepper. Sprinkle any remaining Parmesan mixture over the asparagus.

7. Bake for 20 to 25 minutes, until the pork is cooked through and the coating is crisp.

8. Serve hot.

INGREDIENT TIP: Pork rinds come in a variety of flavors—feel free to experiment to add extra depth to this dish.

Per Batch:
Calories: 740; Total Fat: 42g; Carbs: 12g; Net Carbs: 7g; Fiber: 5g; Protein: 79g

Per Serving:
Calories: 370; Total Fat: 21g; Carbs: 6g; Net Carbs: 4g; Fiber: 3g; Protein: 40g

SESAME PORK AND GREEN BEANS

This quick and flavorful dinner brings bold Asian-inspired flavors to the table in minutes. It's hearty, satisfying, and perfect for a busy night when time is limited but flavor is nonnegotiable.

30-MINUTE
Serves: 2
Prep: 5 minutes
Cook: 10 minutes

Ingredients:

- 2 boneless pork chops
- Pink salt
- Freshly ground black pepper
- 2 tablespoons toasted sesame oil, divided
- 2 tablespoons soy sauce
- 1 teaspoon Sriracha sauce
- 1 cup fresh green beans

Instructions:

1. Pat the pork chops dry with a paper towel. Slice them into thin strips and season with pink salt and pepper.

2. Heat 1 tablespoon of the sesame oil in a large skillet over medium heat.

3. Add the pork strips and cook for about 7 minutes,
   stirring occasionally, until fully cooked and lightly
   browned.

4. In a small bowl, mix the remaining tablespoon of
   sesame oil with the soy sauce and Sriracha. Pour the
   sauce into the skillet.

5. Add the green beans, reduce the heat to
   medium-low, and simmer for 3 to 5 minutes, until
   the beans are tender but still crisp.

6. Divide the pork, green beans, and sauce evenly
   between two wide bowls and serve.

SUBSTITUTION TIP: If Sriracha is too spicy, replace it
with minced fresh ginger for flavor without the heat.

Per Batch:
Calories: 732; Total Fat: 48g; Carbs: 9g; Net Carbs: 6g;
Fiber: 3g; Protein: 65g

Per Serving:
Calories: 366; Total Fat: 24g; Carbs: 5g; Net Carbs: 3g;
Fiber: 2g; Protein: 33g

SLOW-COOKER BARBECUE RIBS

Ribs are a true comfort food, and the slow cooker makes them incredibly easy to prepare. With the help of a good sugar-free barbecue sauce, this recipe delivers tender, flavorful ribs with minimal effort.

ONE POT
Serves: 2
Prep: 10 minutes
Cook: 4 hours

Ingredients:
- 1 pound pork ribs

- Pink salt

- Freshly ground black pepper

- 1 (1.25-ounce) package dry rib seasoning

- ½ cup sugar-free barbecue sauce

Instructions:
1. With the crock insert in place, preheat the slow cooker on high.

2. Season the ribs generously with pink salt, pepper, and the dry rib seasoning.

3. Stand the ribs upright along the inside wall of the slow cooker, with the bone side facing inward.

4. Pour the barbecue sauce over the ribs, using just enough to coat both sides.

5. Cover and cook for 4 hours, until the ribs are tender. Serve carefully.

INGREDIENT TIP: The ribs will be very tender after cooking, so handle them gently when removing them from the slow cooker.

Per Batch:
Calories: 1911; Total Fat: 143g; Carbs: 10g; Net Carbs: 10g; Fiber: 0g; Protein: 136g

Per Serving:
Calories: 956; Total Fat: 72g; Carbs: 5g; Net Carbs: 5g; Fiber: 0g; Protein: 68g

KALUA PORK WITH CABBAGE

After living in Honolulu for nine years, I fell in love with traditional plate lunches—especially kalua pork. While the classic version is served with rice and macaroni salad, this keto-friendly version delivers all the smoky, savory flavor without the carbs.

Serves: 2
Prep: 10 minutes
Cook: 8 hours

Ingredients:

- 1 pound boneless pork butt roast

- Pink salt

- Freshly ground black pepper

- 1 tablespoon smoked paprika or liquid smoke

- ½ cup water

- ½ head cabbage, chopped

Instructions:

1. With the crock insert in place, preheat the slow cooker on low.

2. Season the pork roast generously with pink salt, pepper, and smoked paprika.

3. Place the pork roast into the slow cooker and add the water.

4. Cover and cook on low for 7 hours.

5. Carefully remove the pork roast and place the chopped cabbage in the bottom of the slow cooker. Return the pork to the cooker, placing it on top of the cabbage.

6. Cover and cook for an additional 1 hour, until the cabbage is tender.

7. Remove the pork and place it on a baking sheet. Use two forks to shred the meat.

8. Serve the shredded pork hot alongside the cooked cabbage.

9. Reserve the cooking liquid to moisten leftovers when reheating.

SERVING TIP: Enjoy kalua pork on its own, over cauliflower rice, or on a low-carb roll.

Per Batch:
Calories: 1099; Total Fat: 82g; Carbs: 19g; Net Carbs: 10g; Fiber: 9g; Protein: 77g

Per Serving:
Calories: 550; Total Fat: 41g; Carbs: 10g; Net Carbs: 5g; Fiber: 5g; Protein: 39g

PORK BURGERS WITH SRIRACHA MAYO

Ground pork is often overlooked when it comes to burgers, but it makes incredibly juicy and flavorful patties. In this recipe, fresh scallions and toasted sesame oil add depth to the pork, while a simple Sriracha mayo brings a bold, spicy finish. Enjoy these burgers with a knife and fork or wrapped in crisp lettuce leaves for a perfect keto-friendly meal.

30-MINUTE
SERVES 2
PREP 10 minutes
COOK 10 minutes

Ingredients
12 ounces ground pork
2 scallions (white and green parts), thinly sliced
1 tablespoon toasted sesame oil
Pink salt
Freshly ground black pepper
1 tablespoon ghee
1 tablespoon Sriracha sauce
2 tablespoons mayonnaise

Directions

1. In a large bowl, combine the ground pork, sliced scallions, and sesame oil. Season generously with pink salt and black pepper.
2. Divide the mixture into two equal portions and shape into patties. Press a small indentation into the

center of each patty with your thumb to help the burgers cook evenly.

3. Heat a large skillet over medium-high heat and add the ghee. Once melted and hot, place the patties in the skillet.
4. Cook the burgers for about 4 minutes per side, until browned and cooked through.
5. While the burgers cook, stir together the Sriracha sauce and mayonnaise in a small bowl.
6. Transfer the cooked burgers to a plate and let them rest for at least 5 minutes.
7. Spoon the Sriracha mayo over each burger and serve.

Ingredient Tip
Sriracha can be quite spicy, so adjust the amount to suit your heat preference.

BLUE CHEESE PORK CHOPS

This rich and creamy blue cheese sauce pairs beautifully with pork chops. It comes together quickly and uses simple, keto-friendly ingredients, making it perfect for a fast yet indulgent meal.

30-MINUTE
SERVES 2
PREP 5 minutes
COOK 10 minutes

Ingredients
2 boneless pork chops
Pink salt
Freshly ground black pepper
2 tablespoons butter
⅓ cup blue cheese crumbles

⅓ cup heavy (whipping) cream
⅓ cup sour cream

Directions

1. Pat the pork chops dry with paper towels and season both sides with pink salt and black pepper.
2. Heat a medium skillet over medium heat and melt the butter. Once hot, add the pork chops.
3. Sear the pork chops for about 3 minutes per side, until golden brown. Transfer to a plate and let rest for 3 to 5 minutes.
4. In a medium saucepan over medium heat, add the blue cheese crumbles. Stir frequently until the cheese begins to melt.
5. Add the heavy cream and sour cream, stirring to combine. Let the sauce gently simmer for a few minutes until smooth.
6. For extra flavor, pour the reserved pan juices from the pork chops into the sauce and stir well.
7. Place the pork chops on two plates, spoon the blue cheese sauce generously over the top, and serve.

Ingredient Tip
This blue cheese sauce is also excellent over roasted vegetables.

CARNITAS

Carnitas are ideal for meal prep and make quick, flavorful meals throughout the week. Cooking the pork low and slow allows it to absorb the flavors of garlic, onion, and lime, resulting in tender, shredded meat.

SERVES 2
PREP 10 minutes
COOK 8 hours

Ingredients
½ tablespoon chili powder
1 tablespoon olive oil
1 pound boneless pork butt roast
2 garlic cloves, minced
½ small onion, diced
Pinch pink salt
Pinch freshly ground black pepper
Juice of 1 lime

Directions

1. With the crock insert in place, set the slow cooker to low.
2. In a small bowl, mix the chili powder and olive oil to form a paste. Rub the mixture all over the pork roast.
3. Place the pork roast in the slow cooker, fat-side up.
4. Sprinkle the garlic, onion, pink salt, and black pepper over the pork, then drizzle with lime juice.
5. Cover and cook on low for 8 hours, until the pork is tender and easily shredded.

6. Transfer the pork to a cutting board and shred using
   two forks. Serve immediately or reserve for another
   recipe.

Ingredient Tip
Save the cooking juices to drizzle over the pork before
serving or when reheating leftovers.

CARNITAS NACHOS

These pork-rind nachos are my favorite way to use leftover
carnitas. They're crunchy, cheesy, and incredibly
satisfying—without the carbs of traditional nachos.

30-MINUTE
SERVES 2
PREP 5 minutes
COOK 10 minutes

Ingredients
1 tablespoon olive oil, plus more for coating
2 cups pork rinds
½ cup shredded cheese (Mexican blend works well)
1 cup Carnitas
1 avocado, diced
2 tablespoons sour cream

Directions

1. Preheat the oven to 350°F. Lightly coat a
   9-by-13-inch baking dish with olive oil.
2. Spread the pork rinds evenly in the dish and
   sprinkle the shredded cheese over the top.
3. Bake for about 5 minutes, until the cheese has
   melted. Remove from the oven and let rest for 5
   minutes.

4. Heat the olive oil in a medium skillet over high heat. Add the carnitas along with a little of the reserved cooking juice.
5. Cook until the pork develops a crispy crust, then flip and cook briefly on the other side.
6. Divide the cheesy pork rinds between two plates.
7. Top with the crispy carnitas, diced avocado, and a dollop of sour cream. Serve hot.

Ingredient Tip
Watch the cheese closely—it melts quickly and continues melting after removal from the oven.

PEPPERONI LOW-CARB TORTILLA PIZZA

This quick skillet pizza is one of the easiest low-carb dinners you can make. It's perfect for late nights when you want something satisfying without a lot of prep.

30-MINUTE
ONE PAN
SERVES 2
PREP 5 minutes
COOK 5 minutes

Ingredients
2 tablespoons olive oil
2 large low-carb tortillas
4 tablespoons low-sugar tomato sauce
1 cup shredded mozzarella cheese
2 teaspoons dried Italian seasoning
½ cup pepperoni

Directions

1. Heat a medium skillet over medium-high heat and
    add the olive oil.
2. Place one tortilla in the skillet. Quickly spread the
    tomato sauce evenly over the surface.
3. Sprinkle on the mozzarella cheese, Italian
    seasoning, and pepperoni.
4. Cook for about 3 minutes, until the bottom of the
    tortilla is crisp.
5. Transfer to a cutting board, slice, and serve
    immediately.

Ingredient Tip
The olive oil helps the tortilla crisp up, giving it a true
pizza-like texture.

BEEF AND BROCCOLI ROAST

This slow-cooker dish is a simple, keto-friendly take on a
classic favorite. Making it at home ensures full control over
ingredients while delivering rich flavor and tender beef.

SERVES 2
PREP 10 minutes
COOK 4 hours 30 minutes

Ingredients
1 pound beef chuck roast
Pink salt
Freshly ground black pepper
½ cup beef broth, plus more if needed
¼ cup soy sauce (or coconut aminos)
1 teaspoon toasted sesame oil
1 (16-ounce) bag frozen broccoli

Directions

1. With the crock insert in place, set the slow cooker to low.
2. Season the chuck roast with pink salt and pepper, then slice thinly against the grain. Transfer the beef to the slow cooker.
3. In a small bowl, mix the beef broth, soy sauce, and sesame oil. Pour over the beef.
4. Cover and cook on low for 4 hours.
5. Add the frozen broccoli and continue cooking for 30 minutes. Add more broth if additional liquid is needed.
6. Serve hot.

Serving Tip

This dish pairs beautifully with shirataki rice or cauliflower rice.

BEEF AND BELL PEPPER "POTATO SKINS"

This is one of my favorite creative, low-carb spins on classic game-day food. I make pork-rind and cauliflower nachos often, but one day it clicked: thick bell pepper slices make the perfect low-carb "potato skin." They're sturdy enough to hold all the toppings while adding a fresh, crisp bite. The result is colorful, satisfying, and endlessly customizable.

30-MINUTE
SERVES 2
PREP: 10 minutes
COOK: 20 minutes

Ingredients

- 1 tablespoon ghee

- ½ pound ground beef

- Pink salt

- Freshly ground black pepper

- 3 large bell peppers (use different colors if possible)

- ½ cup shredded cheese (Mexican blend recommended)

- 1 avocado

- ¼ cup sour cream

Instructions

1. Preheat the oven to 400°F. Line a baking sheet with aluminum foil or a silicone baking mat for easy cleanup.

2. In a large skillet over medium-high heat, melt the ghee. Once hot, add the ground beef. Season with pink salt and black pepper. Cook for 7 to 10 minutes, stirring occasionally and breaking the meat apart, until fully browned. Remove from heat.

3. While the beef cooks, prepare the bell peppers. Slice off the tops, cut each pepper in half, and remove the seeds and ribs. If the peppers are very large, cut them into quarters so each piece resembles a potato-skin-sized "boat."

4. Arrange the pepper pieces cut-side up on the prepared baking sheet.

5. Spoon the cooked ground beef evenly into each pepper piece. Sprinkle shredded cheese generously over the top.

6. Bake for 10 minutes, or until the peppers are slightly tender and the cheese is fully melted.

7. While the peppers bake, prepare the avocado crema by combining the avocado and sour cream in a medium bowl. Mash and mix until smooth.

8. Remove the peppers from the oven. Divide between two plates, top with the avocado crema, and serve warm.

SUBSTITUTION TIP: Ground turkey works well in place of ground beef.

Per Batch:
Calories: 1413; Total Fat: 103g; Carbs: 44g; Net Carbs: 25g; Fiber: 19g; Protein: 80g

Per Serving:
Calories: 707; Total Fat: 52g; Carbs: 22g; Net Carbs: 13g; Fiber: 10g; Protein: 40g

SKIRT STEAK WITH CHIMICHURRI SAUCE

This dish delivers bold, savory flavor with minimal effort. The key is allowing enough time for the steak to marinate, which makes it incredibly tender. Once seared, the steak is sliced thin and topped with a garlicky chimichurri sauce that instantly wakes up your taste buds.

SERVES 2
PREP: 10 minutes, plus marinating time
COOK: 10 minutes

Ingredients
- ½ cup soy sauce
- ½ cup olive oil
- Juice of 1 lime
- 2 tablespoons apple cider vinegar
- 1 pound skirt steak
- Pink salt
- Freshly ground black pepper
- 2 tablespoons ghee
- ½ cup chimichurri sauce

Instructions
1. In a small bowl, whisk together the soy sauce, olive oil, lime juice, and apple cider vinegar.

2. Pour the marinade into a large zip-top bag. Add the skirt steak, seal, and refrigerate for at least all day, preferably overnight.

3. Remove the steak from the marinade and pat completely dry with paper towels. Season both sides with pink salt and black pepper.

4. Heat a large skillet over high heat and melt the ghee. Once very hot, add the steak and sear for about 4 minutes per side, until deeply browned.

5. Transfer the steak to a cutting board and allow it to rest for at least 5 minutes.

6. Slice the steak thinly against the grain. Divide between two plates, top with chimichurri sauce, and serve.

INGREDIENT TIP: Homemade chimichurri can be made with cilantro, parsley, red onion, garlic, olive oil, apple cider vinegar, salt, and pepper.

Per Batch:
Calories: 1435; Total Fat: 91g; Carbs: 12g; Net Carbs: 8g; Fiber: 4g; Protein: 139g

Per Serving:
Calories: 718; Total Fat: 46g; Carbs: 6g; Net Carbs: 4g; Fiber: 2g; Protein: 70g

BARBACOA BEEF ROAST

Inspired by my love for Chipotle's barbacoa, this slow-cooker version delivers incredible flavor with just five ingredients. After eight hours, the beef becomes melt-in-your-mouth tender and shreds effortlessly.

SERVES 2
PREP: 10 minutes
COOK: 8 hours

Instructions

1. Preheat the slow cooker to low.

2. Season the beef chuck roast generously with pink salt and black pepper. Place it in the slow cooker.

3. In a food processor or blender, combine the chipotle peppers with adobo sauce, jalapeños, and apple cider vinegar. Blend until smooth, then add the beef broth and pulse briefly.

4. Pour the sauce over the beef.

5. Cover and cook on low for 8 hours.

6. Transfer the beef to a cutting board and shred using two forks. Serve hot.

INGREDIENT TIP: Beef brisket can be used instead of chuck roast.

STEAK AND EGG BIBIMBAP

Bibimbap means "mixed rice" in Korean, and while this version isn't traditional, it keeps the heart of the dish intact: savory beef, a runny egg, and crisp vegetables. This is a great recipe for using up leftovers, and it comes together quickly with minimal prep.

30-MINUTE
SERVES 2
PREP: 10 minutes
COOK: 15 minutes

Ingredients
FOR THE GROUND BEEF

- 1 tablespoon ghee

- ½ pound ground beef or finely minced steak

- Pink salt

- Freshly ground black pepper

- 1 tablespoon soy sauce (or coconut aminos)

FOR THE EGG AND CAULIFLOWER RICE

- 2 tablespoons ghee, divided

- 2 large eggs

- 1 large cucumber, peeled and cut into matchsticks

- 1 tablespoon soy sauce

- 1 cup cauliflower rice

- Pink salt

- Freshly ground black pepper

Instructions
To Make the Ground Beef
1. Heat a large skillet over medium-high heat and add the ghee.

2. When the ghee is hot, add the ground beef. Season with pink salt and black pepper.

3. Cook for about 7 to 8 minutes, stirring occasionally and breaking the meat apart with a wooden spoon, until fully browned.

4. Add the soy sauce, stir well, then reduce the heat to medium-low and allow the beef to simmer gently while you prepare the remaining components.

To Make the Egg and Cauliflower Rice
1. In a second large skillet over medium-high heat, heat 1 tablespoon of ghee.

2. Once hot, crack the eggs directly into the pan. Cook for 2 to 3 minutes, until the whites are set but the yolks remain runny. Carefully transfer the eggs to a plate.

3. Place the cucumber matchsticks in a small bowl and toss with the soy sauce. Set aside to lightly marinate.

4. Wipe out the skillet used for the eggs, then return it to the heat and add the remaining 1 tablespoon of ghee.

5. Add the cauliflower rice to the skillet. Season with pink salt and black pepper and cook, stirring occasionally, for about 5 minutes.

6. Increase the heat to high during the final minute to give the cauliflower rice a lightly crisp texture.

7. Divide the cauliflower rice evenly between two bowls.

8. Top each bowl with the ground beef, a fried egg, and the marinated cucumber. Serve immediately.

VARIATIONS

- Kimchi

- Sriracha drizzled on top

- Bean sprouts

- Carrot matchsticks

- Chopped mushrooms

- Chopped scallions

INGREDIENT TIP: Ground turkey can be used in place of ground beef.

MISSISSIPPI POT ROAST

This slow-cooker favorite is one of the most requested recipes on my keto feed. It's incredibly simple, packed with flavor, and practically cooks itself. The pepperoncini add a tangy kick that balances the richness of the meat beautifully.

ONE POT
SERVES 4
PREP: 5 minutes
COOK: 8 hours

Ingredients

- 1 pound beef chuck roast

- Pink salt

- Freshly ground black pepper

- 1 (1-ounce) packet dry au jus gravy mix

- 1 (1-ounce) packet dry ranch dressing mix

- 8 tablespoons butter (1 stick)

- 1 cup whole pepperoncini

Instructions

1. Preheat the slow cooker to low.

2. Season both sides of the beef chuck roast generously with pink salt and black pepper.

3. Place the roast in the slow cooker.

4. Sprinkle the au jus gravy mix and ranch dressing mix evenly over the top of the roast.

5. Place the stick of butter directly on top of the meat.

6. Scatter the pepperoncini around the roast.

7. Cover and cook on low for 8 hours.

8. Remove the roast from the slow cooker and shred the meat using two forks.

9. Serve hot with the cooking juices spooned over the top if desired.

INGREDIENT TIP: This recipe also works beautifully with boneless chicken breasts.

TACO CHEESE CUPS

These crunchy cheese cups are fun to make and incredibly versatile. Once you master the technique, you'll want to use them for everything—from tacos to salads to snack bowls.

30-MINUTE
SERVES 2
PREP: 10 minutes
COOK: 20 minutes

Ingredients
FOR THE CHEESE CUPS

- 2 cups shredded cheese (Mexican blend recommended)

FOR THE GROUND BEEF

- 1 tablespoon ghee

- ½ pound ground beef

- ½ (1.25-ounce) packet taco seasoning

- ¼ cup water

FOR ASSEMBLY

- ½ avocado, diced

- Pink salt

- Freshly ground black pepper

- 2 tablespoons sour cream

Instructions

To Make the Cheese Cups

1. Preheat the oven to 350°F. Line a baking sheet with parchment paper or a silicone baking mat.

2. Place ½-cup mounds of shredded cheese on the prepared baking sheet, spacing them apart.

3. Bake for about 7 minutes, until the edges are golden brown and the centers are fully melted.

4. Remove the pan from the oven and let the cheese cool for 2 minutes. The cheese will still be flexible.

5. Carefully transfer each cheese round into a muffin tin, gently pressing it into the cup to form a bowl shape.

6. Allow the cheese cups to cool completely in the muffin tin until firm.

To Make the Ground Beef

1. Heat a medium skillet over medium-high heat and add the ghee.

2. When hot, add the ground beef and cook for about 8 minutes, stirring and breaking it apart until browned.

3. Drain excess grease.

4. Stir in the taco seasoning and water. Bring to a boil, then reduce heat and simmer for 5 minutes.

To Assemble

1. Spoon the ground beef into each cheese cup using a slotted spoon.

2. Season the diced avocado with pink salt and black pepper and divide among the cups.

3. Add a dollop of sour cream to each and serve immediately.

BACON CHEESEBURGER CASSEROLE

This hearty, protein-packed casserole reheats beautifully and is perfect for busy weeks. It's rich, filling, and a family favorite in my house.

SERVES 4
PREP: 10 minutes
COOK: 50 minutes

Instructions
To Make the Bacon and Ground Beef
1. In a large skillet over medium-high heat, cook the bacon until crispy, about 8 minutes. Transfer to a paper towel–lined plate to cool, then chop.

2. In a second skillet, heat the ghee over medium-high heat.

3. Add the ground beef, season with pink salt and black pepper, and cook for about 8 minutes, breaking it apart until browned.

4. Drain excess fat and stir in the chopped bacon.

To Make the Casserole
1. Preheat the oven to 350°F. Grease a 9-by-13-inch baking dish with ghee.

2. Spread the meat-and-bacon mixture evenly in the dish.

3. In a medium bowl, whisk together the cream, eggs, and half of the shredded cheese. Season with pink salt and black pepper.

4. Pour the egg mixture over the meat. Sprinkle the
   remaining cheese on top.

5. Bake for 30 minutes, until the cheese is melted and
   lightly browned.

6. Let rest for 5 minutes before slicing and serving.

FETA-STUFFED BURGERS

These juicy burgers combine beef and lamb with fresh herbs and a creamy feta center for a Mediterranean-inspired keto meal.

30-MINUTE
SERVES 2
PREP: 10 minutes
COOK: 10 minutes

Instructions

1. In a large bowl, combine the chopped mint, scallion, and Dijon mustard. Season with pink salt and black pepper.

2. Add the ground beef and lamb mixture. Mix thoroughly until evenly combined.

3. Divide the mixture into 4 equal patties.

4. Press the feta cheese into the center of 2 patties. Top each with another patty and pinch the edges tightly to seal in the cheese.

5. Heat a skillet over medium heat and add the ghee.

6. Cook the burgers for 4 to 5 minutes per side, until cooked to your preferred doneness.

7. Serve hot.

CHAPTER SEVEN
DESSERTS & SWEET TREATS

Desserts can absolutely be fun on a keto diet! I like to keep my dessert recipes simple, so when a sweet craving hits, I can whip something up quickly using ingredients I already have at home. I usually enjoy dessert as an occasional treat, maybe once a week, because I find that the less I eat sweets, the less I crave them. These recipes focus on just five ingredients or fewer, making keto desserts both easy and satisfying.

Blueberry-Blackberry Ice Pops
Strawberry-Lime Ice Pops
Coffee Ice Pops
Fudge Ice Pops
Root Beer Float
Orange Cream Float
Strawberry Shake
"Frosty" Chocolate Shake
Strawberry Cheesecake Mousse
Lemonade Fat Bomb
Berry Cheesecake Fat Bomb
Peanut Butter Fat Bomb
Crustless Cheesecake Bites
Pumpkin Crustless Cheesecake Bites
Berry-Pecan Mascarpone Bowl
Peanut Butter Cookies
Chocolate Mousse
Mint–Chocolate Chip Ice Cream
Chocolate-Avocado Pudding

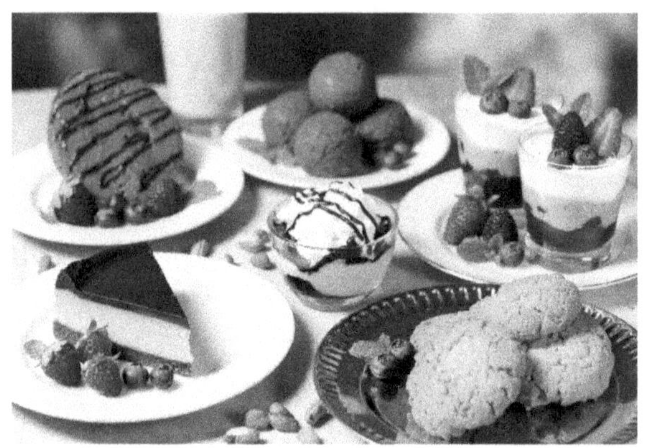

BLUEBERRY-BLACKBERRY ICE POPS

Blueberries are my favorite fruit, and blackberries come in a close second. I created this creamy, refreshing ice pop using both, and the color is absolutely gorgeous!

No Cook | Vegetarian
Serves 2
Prep: 5 minutes + at least 2 hours to freeze

Ingredients
- ½ (13.5-ounce) can coconut cream, or ¾ cup unsweetened full-fat coconut milk, or ¾ cup heavy (whipping) cream

- 2 teaspoons Swerve natural sweetener, or 2 drops liquid stevia

- ½ teaspoon vanilla extract

- ¼ cup mixed blueberries and blackberries (fresh or frozen)

Instructions
1. In a food processor or blender, combine the coconut cream, sweetener, and vanilla extract.

2. Add the mixed berries and pulse a few times, just enough to keep the blueberries' texture intact.

3. Pour the mixture into ice pop molds and freeze for at least 2 hours before serving.

Ingredient Tip: If you don't have both blueberries and blackberries, feel free to use just one or the other.

Nutrition per Serving:
Calories: 165 | Total Fat: 17g | Carbs: 4g | Net Carbs: 2g | Fiber: 1g | Protein: 1g

STRAWBERRY-LIME ICE POPS

This ice pop reminds me of a fresh Mexican paleta, with the perfect balance of sweet, creamy, and sour flavors thanks to the lime juice.

No Cook | Vegetarian
Serves 4
Prep: 5 minutes + at least 2 hours to freeze

Ingredients
- ½ (13.5-ounce) can coconut cream, or ¾ cup unsweetened full-fat coconut milk, or ¾ cup heavy (whipping) cream

- 2 teaspoons Swerve natural sweetener, or 2 drops liquid stevia

- 1 tablespoon freshly squeezed lime juice

- ¼ cup hulled and sliced strawberries (fresh or frozen)

Instructions
1. In a food processor or blender, combine the coconut cream, sweetener, and lime juice.

2. Add the strawberries and pulse a few times so they keep some texture.

3. Pour into ice pop molds and freeze for at least 2 hours before serving.

Ingredient Tip: You can substitute blackberries for strawberries if you prefer.

Nutrition per Serving:
Calories: 166 | Total Fat: 17g | Carbs: 5g | Net Carbs: 3g | Fiber: 1g | Protein: 1g

COFFEE ICE POPS

Coffee lovers on keto will enjoy these convenient frozen treats. The rich blend of coffee and cream gets an extra touch of fun with sugar-free chocolate chips.

No Cook | Vegetarian
Serves 4
Prep: 5 minutes + 2 hours to freeze

Ingredients
- 2 cups brewed coffee, cold

- ¾ cup coconut cream, or unsweetened full-fat coconut milk, or heavy (whipping) cream

- 2 teaspoons Swerve natural sweetener, or 2 drops liquid stevia

- 2 tablespoons sugar-free chocolate chips (I use Lily's)

Instructions
1. In a food processor or blender, blend together the coffee, coconut cream, and sweetener until smooth.

2. Pour the mixture into ice pop molds, then drop a few chocolate chips into each mold.

3. Freeze for at least 2 hours before serving.

Variations:
Customize your coffee ice pops with your favorite sugar-free flavorings, such as:

- Cinnamon

- Vanilla

- Chocolate protein powder

Ingredient Tip: Adjust the sweetness to your personal preference.

Nutrition per Serving:
Calories: 105 | Total Fat: 10g | Carbs: 7g | Net Carbs: 2g | Fiber: 2g | Protein: 1g

FUDGE ICE POPS

I love fudge ice pops because they're simple to make and satisfy sweet cravings instantly. They're also a great canvas for creative flavors. Investing in quality ice pop molds really pays off!

No Cook | Vegetarian
Serves 4
Prep: 5 minutes + 2 hours to freeze

Ingredients
- ½ (13.5-ounce) can coconut cream, or ¾ cup unsweetened full-fat coconut milk, or ¾ cup heavy (whipping) cream

- 2 teaspoons Swerve natural sweetener, or 2 drops liquid stevia

- 2 tablespoons unsweetened cocoa powder

- 2 tablespoons sugar-free chocolate chips (I use Lily's)

Instructions
1. In a food processor or blender, combine the coconut cream, sweetener, and cocoa powder until smooth.

2. Pour the mixture into ice pop molds and add chocolate chips to each mold.

3. Freeze for at least 2 hours before serving.

Variations:

- Add collagen powder for extra health benefits.

- Use heavy cream and fold in cream cheese for a richer texture, then add chocolate chips last.

Ingredient Tip: Feel free to adjust the sweetness to your liking.

Nutrition per Serving:
Calories: 193 | Total Fat: 20g | Carbs: 9g | Net Carbs: 3g | Fiber: 3g | Protein: 2g

ROOT BEER FLOAT

Discover how easy it is to make a keto-friendly root beer float! This creamy, fizzy treat is delicious and sugar-free — you won't miss the sugar at all.

30-Minute | One Pan | No Cook | Vegetarian
Serves 2
Prep: 5 minutes

Ingredients
- 1 (12-ounce) can diet root beer (I like Zevia's)

- 4 tablespoons heavy (whipping) cream

- 1 teaspoon vanilla extract

- 6 ice cubes

Instructions
1. In a food processor or blender, combine the root beer, heavy cream, vanilla extract, and ice cubes.

2. Blend until smooth and frothy.

3. Pour into two tall glasses and serve immediately.

Ingredient Tip: For a boozy twist, add vanilla vodka or rum.

Nutrition per Serving:
Calories: 56 | Total Fat: 6g | Carbs: 3g | Net Carbs: 1g | Fiber: 0g | Protein: 1g

ORANGE CREAM FLOAT

Orange flavor is a rare delight on keto, so I was excited to discover Zevia's Orange Soda, sweetened with stevia. This float is creamy, tangy, and refreshing.

30-Minute | One Pan | No Cook | Vegetarian
Serves 2
Prep: 5 minutes

Ingredients
- 1 can diet orange soda (I like Zevia's)
- 4 tablespoons heavy (whipping) cream
- 1 teaspoon vanilla extract
- 6 ice cubes

Instructions
1. In a food processor or blender, combine the orange soda, heavy cream, vanilla extract, and ice cubes.
2. Blend until smooth and creamy.
3. Pour into two tall glasses and serve immediately.

Ingredient Tip: Add vanilla vodka for an adult version of this treat.

Nutrition per Serving:
Calories: 56 | Total Fat: 6g | Carbs: 3g | Net Carbs: 1g |
Fiber: 0g | Protein: 1g

STRAWBERRY SHAKE

If you've noticed by now, I absolutely love cheesecake —
so why not enjoy a strawberry cheesecake–inspired shake?
No baking or waiting around, just a quick blend and you're
ready to enjoy!

30-Minute | One Pan | No Cook | Vegetarian
Serves 2
Prep: 10 minutes

Ingredients

- ¾ cup heavy (whipping) cream

- 2 ounces cream cheese, softened to room
  temperature

- 1 tablespoon Swerve natural sweetener

- ¼ teaspoon vanilla extract

- 6 strawberries, sliced

- 6 ice cubes

Instructions

1. In a food processor or blender, combine the heavy
   cream, cream cheese, sweetener, and vanilla extract.
   Blend on high until fully combined and smooth.

2. Add the sliced strawberries and ice cubes, then
   blend again until smooth and creamy.

3. Pour into two tall glasses and serve immediately.

Ingredient Tip: A swirl of whipped cream on top adds an extra-special touch to any milkshake!

"FROSTY" CHOCOLATE SHAKE

I used to love indulging in Frostys before keto, and this copycat recipe gets remarkably close to the real deal. I use coconut milk straight from a 13.5-ounce can stirred well after opening. For best results, chill a metal mixing bowl and your mixer beaters in the freezer before starting.

One Pan | No Cook | Vegetarian
Serves 2
Prep: 10 minutes + 1 hour chill

Ingredients
- ¾ cup heavy (whipping) cream
- 4 ounces coconut milk (full-fat)
- 1 tablespoon Swerve natural sweetener
- ¼ teaspoon vanilla extract
- 2 tablespoons unsweetened cocoa powder

Instructions
1. Pour the heavy cream into the chilled metal bowl. Using cold beaters on a hand mixer, whip the cream just until it forms soft peaks.

2. Slowly add the coconut milk, gently folding it into the whipped cream. Then add the sweetener, vanilla extract, and cocoa powder. Beat until everything is fully combined and smooth.

3. Pour the shake into two tall glasses, then chill in the freezer for 1 hour before serving. During this time, I

like to stir the shake twice to keep the texture smooth.

Ingredient Tip: If you don't have coconut milk, almond milk is a fine substitute.

STRAWBERRY CHEESECAKE MOUSSE

This mousse is a super-easy, no-bake cheesecake treat that any cheesecake fan will devour! Ready in 10 minutes and customizable with your favorite fruits.

One Pan | No Cook | Vegetarian
Serves 2
Prep: 10 minutes + 1 hour chill

Ingredients
- 4 ounces cream cheese, softened to room temperature

- 1 tablespoon heavy (whipping) cream

- 1 teaspoon Swerve natural sweetener, or 1 drop liquid stevia

- 1 teaspoon vanilla extract

- 4 strawberries, sliced (fresh or frozen)

Instructions
1. Break the cream cheese into smaller chunks and add to a food processor or blender. Add the heavy cream, sweetener, and vanilla extract.

2. Blend on high, stopping occasionally to scrape down the sides, until smooth and well combined.

3. Add the sliced strawberries, and pulse briefly to incorporate them into the mousse.

4. Divide the mousse evenly into two small serving dishes and chill in the refrigerator for 1 hour before serving.

Variations:

- Swap strawberries for about ¼ cup blackberries.

- For a festive twist during winter, substitute 3 ounces pumpkin purée and add 1 teaspoon pumpkin pie spice instead of strawberries.

Ingredient Tip: The heavy cream helps soften the cream cheese. If the mixture feels too thick, add a little more cream while blending.

LEMONADE FAT BOMB

Fat bombs are a keto staple, and this lemonade version is a favorite in my family — especially with my lemon-loving daughter! For best results, let all ingredients sit at room temperature for about 2 hours before starting.

No Cook | Vegetarian
Serves 2
Prep: 10 minutes + 2 hours freeze

Ingredients
- Zest of ½ lemon (using a fine grater)

- Juice of ½ lemon

- 4 ounces cream cheese, softened to room temperature

- 2 ounces butter, softened to room temperature

- 2 teaspoons Swerve natural sweetener or 2 drops liquid stevia

- Pinch of pink salt

Instructions
1. In a small bowl, combine the lemon zest and juice.

2. In a medium bowl, beat together the cream cheese and butter with a hand mixer until smooth. Add the sweetener, lemon mixture, and pink salt, and beat until fully combined.

3. Spoon the mixture into fat bomb molds — I like using small silicone cupcake molds placed in a muffin tin. If you don't have molds, cupcake liners work well too.

4. Freeze for at least 2 hours until firm. Unmold and enjoy! Keep extras stored in a zip-top bag in the freezer for up to 3 months.

Cooking Tip: An ice cube tray makes a simple and effective mold for fat bombs.

BERRY CHEESECAKE FAT BOMB

These fat bombs deliver all the rich flavor of cheesecake in a small, satisfying bite. I love using a mix of strawberries and blackberries, mashed together before folding in. As with all fat bombs, ingredients should be at room temperature for the best texture.

No Cook | Vegetarian
Serves 2
Prep: 10 minutes + at least 2 hours freeze

Ingredients
- 4 ounces cream cheese, softened to room temperature

- 4 tablespoons (½ stick) butter, softened to room temperature

- 2 teaspoons Swerve natural sweetener or 2 drops liquid stevia

- 1 teaspoon vanilla extract

- ¼ cup berries (fresh or frozen)

Instructions
1. In a medium bowl, beat the cream cheese, butter, sweetener, and vanilla with a hand mixer until smooth.

2. In a small bowl, mash the berries thoroughly. Fold the mashed berries gently into the cream cheese mixture with a rubber spatula. (Avoid adding whole berry slices as they can freeze and affect texture.)

3. Spoon the mixture into fat bomb molds or cupcake liners placed in a muffin tin.

4. Freeze for at least 2 hours until firm. Unmold and serve! Store leftovers in the freezer in a zip-top bag for up to 3 months.

Cooking Tip: Use an ice cube tray for a quick and easy fat bomb mold.

PEANUT BUTTER FAT BOMB

These peanut butter fat bombs are a quick, kid-approved treat — perfect for making ahead while you prepare dinner. Again, ingredients should be at room temperature for smooth mixing.

Vegetarian
Serves 2
Prep: 10 minutes + 30 minutes freeze

Ingredients
- 1 tablespoon butter, softened to room temperature

- 1 tablespoon coconut oil

- 2 tablespoons all-natural peanut butter or almond butter

- 2 teaspoons Swerve natural sweetener or 2 drops liquid stevia

Instructions

1. In a microwave-safe medium bowl, melt the butter, coconut oil, and peanut butter on 50% power in the microwave until fully melted. Stir in the sweetener.

2. Pour the mixture into fat bomb molds — I use small silicone cupcake molds.

3. Freeze for 30 minutes until firm. Unmold and enjoy! Keep extras stored in the freezer in a zip-top bag for up to 3 months.

Cooking Tip: An ice cube tray works well as a fat bomb mold. After freezing, pop them out, store in a bag, and keep frozen.

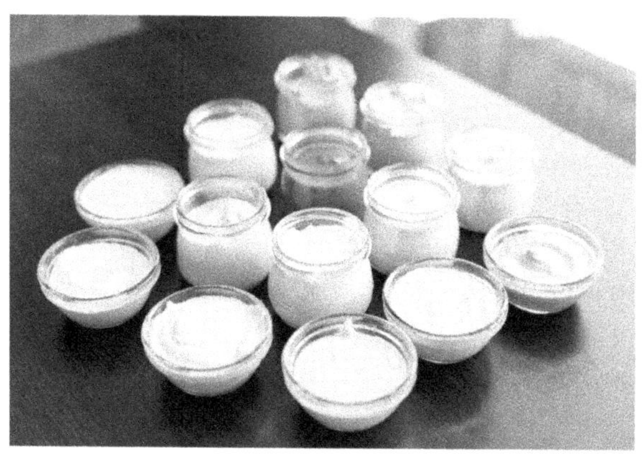

CHAPTER EIGHT
SAUCES & DRESSINGS

When following a low-carb lifestyle, having delicious sauces and dressings on hand can truly elevate any meal. While there are plenty of great store-bought options, making your own at home offers unbeatable benefits. Not only do you control every ingredient, ensuring quality and freshness, but you also manage exactly how many carbs go into your dishes.

The recipes in this chapter are some of my personal favorites — simple, flavorful, and mostly made from ingredients you likely already have in your fridge or pantry. Whether you're looking to brighten up a salad, add richness to grilled meats, or spice up a snack, these homemade sauces and dressings will make your meals both healthier and more delicious.

DIJON VINAIGRETTE

A light, tangy dressing that beautifully complements salads featuring tomatoes, berries, or other sweet elements. The sharpness of Dijon mustard balances the flavors perfectly.

30-Minute | One Pan | No Cook | Vegetarian
Serves 4
Prep: 5 minutes

Ingredients:

- 2 tablespoons Dijon mustard
- Juice of ½ lemon
- 1 garlic clove, finely minced
- 1½ tablespoons red wine vinegar
- Pink salt, to taste
- Freshly ground black pepper, to taste
- 3 tablespoons olive oil

Instructions:

1. In a small bowl, whisk together the Dijon mustard, lemon juice, minced garlic, and red wine vinegar until well combined.
2. Season with pink salt and freshly ground black pepper, then whisk again to incorporate.
3. Slowly drizzle in the olive oil while whisking constantly to emulsify the dressing.
4. Transfer the vinaigrette to a sealed glass container and refrigerate. It will keep for up to one week.

Substitution Tip: You can substitute red wine vinegar with apple cider vinegar if preferred.

GREEN GODDESS DRESSING

This creamy, fresh dressing comes together quickly and adds a burst of flavor to salads or grilled meats. It pairs wonderfully with grilled beef or chicken.

30-Minute | One Pot | No Cook | Vegetarian
Serves 4
Prep: 5 minutes

Ingredients:

- 2 tablespoons buttermilk
- ¼ cup Greek yogurt
- 1 teaspoon apple cider vinegar
- 1 garlic clove, minced
- 1 tablespoon olive oil
- 1 tablespoon fresh parsley leaves

Instructions:

1. Combine buttermilk, Greek yogurt, apple cider vinegar, minced garlic, olive oil, and parsley in a food processor or blender.
2. Blend until smooth and fully combined.
3. Pour the dressing into a sealed container and chill for at least 30 minutes to let the flavors meld.
4. Store in the refrigerator for up to one week.

Substitution Tip: You can replace Greek yogurt with sour cream, or add fresh chopped chives with the parsley for extra flavor.

CAESAR DRESSING

A keto-friendly classic, rich in healthy fats and savory flavor, perfect for elevating even the simplest salad.

30-Minute | One Pan | No Cook
Serves 4
Prep: 5 minutes

Ingredients:

- ½ cup mayonnaise
- 1 tablespoon Dijon mustard
- Juice of ½ lemon
- ½ teaspoon Worcestershire sauce
- Pinch of pink salt
- Pinch of freshly ground black pepper
- ¼ cup grated Parmesan cheese

Instructions:

1. Whisk together mayonnaise, Dijon mustard, lemon juice, Worcestershire sauce, pink salt, and black pepper in a medium bowl until smooth and well blended.
2. Stir in grated Parmesan cheese until creamy.
3. Store in a sealed container in the refrigerator for up to one week.

Variations:

- Add 1 teaspoon anchovy paste for a traditional Caesar flavor.
- Mix in ¼ cup sour cream and minced garlic for added tang and depth.

Storage Tip: Mason jars are ideal for storing homemade dressings.

AVOCADO-LIME CREMA

A smooth, creamy sauce reminiscent of guacamole, perfect for topping salads, tacos, and meat dishes.

30-Minute | One Pot | No Cook | Vegetarian
Serves 4
Prep: 5 minutes

Ingredients:

- ½ cup sour cream
- ½ avocado
- 1 garlic clove, finely minced
- ¼ cup fresh cilantro leaves
- Juice of ½ lime
- Pinch of pink salt
- Pinch of freshly ground black pepper

Instructions:

1. In a food processor or blender, combine sour cream, avocado, garlic, cilantro, lime juice, pink salt, and black pepper.
2. Blend until smooth and fully combined.
3. Transfer to an airtight jar and refrigerate for up to 3 days.

Serving Tip: For a beautiful presentation, put the crema in a zip-top bag and cut a small corner to pipe it over tacos, deviled eggs, or grilled meats.

CHUNKY BLUE CHEESE DRESSING

Perfect for wedge salads, steak salads, or as a dip for crispy hot wings—rich, creamy, and packed with blue cheese flavor.

30-Minute | One Pan | No Cook
Serves 4
Prep: 5 minutes

Ingredients:

- ½ cup sour cream
- ½ cup mayonnaise
- Juice of ½ lemon
- ½ teaspoon Worcestershire sauce
- Pink salt, to taste
- Freshly ground black pepper, to taste
- 2 ounces crumbled blue cheese

Instructions:

1. In a medium bowl, whisk together sour cream, mayonnaise, lemon juice, and Worcestershire sauce. Season with pink salt and pepper, then whisk again until smooth.
2. Fold in the crumbled blue cheese, adjusting the amount based on how chunky you like your dressing.
3. Store in a sealed container in the refrigerator for up to one week.

SRIRACHA MAYO

Creamy and spicy, this sauce adds a kick to chicken, veggies, and more — a quick and versatile condiment.

30-Minute | One Pan | No Cook | Vegetarian
Serves 4
Prep: 5 minutes

Ingredients:

- ½ cup mayonnaise
- 2 tablespoons Sriracha sauce
- ½ teaspoon garlic powder
- ½ teaspoon onion powder
- ¼ teaspoon paprika

Instructions:

1. In a small bowl, whisk together mayonnaise, Sriracha, garlic powder, onion powder, and paprika until well combined.
2. Transfer to an airtight container and refrigerate for up to one week.

Spice Tip: Adjust the amount of Sriracha to control the heat level.

AVOCADO MAYO

Making your own mayonnaise using avocado is simple and delicious. Whether you're out of store-bought mayo or just enjoy crafting your own, this avocado mayo is perfect for mixing into dishes or topping a keto-friendly burger or sandwich.

30-Minute | One Pan | No Cook | Vegetarian
Serves: 4
Prep: 5 minutes

Ingredients:
- 1 medium avocado, cut into chunks

- ½ teaspoon ground cayenne pepper

- Juice of ½ lime

- 2 tablespoons fresh cilantro leaves (optional)

- Pinch of pink salt

- ¼ cup olive oil

Instructions:
1. In a food processor or blender, combine the avocado, cayenne pepper, lime juice, cilantro (if using), and pink salt. Blend until smooth and fully combined.

2. Slowly add the olive oil, about 1 tablespoon at a time, pulsing the processor between additions to incorporate the oil evenly.

3. Transfer to a sealed glass container and store in the refrigerator for up to 1 week.

Ingredient Tip:
Choose an avocado that yields gently to light thumb pressure near the stem—ripe but not overly soft or hard.

Nutrition (Per Serving):
Calories: 58 | Fat: 5g | Carbs: 4g | Net Carbs: 1g | Fiber: 3g | Protein: 1g

PEANUT SAUCE

Peanut sauce adds a rich, nutty flavor that transforms chicken dishes and pairs beautifully with zoodles or any meal where you want an Asian-inspired kick.

30-Minute | One Pan | No Cook | Vegetarian
Serves: 4
Prep: 5 minutes

Ingredients:

- ½ cup creamy peanut butter (Justin's recommended)

- 2 tablespoons soy sauce (or coconut aminos)

- 1 teaspoon Sriracha sauce

- 1 teaspoon toasted sesame oil

- 1 teaspoon garlic powder

Instructions:

1. Combine all ingredients in a food processor or blender. Blend until the sauce is smooth and well mixed.

2. Pour into an airtight container and refrigerate for up to 1 week.

Ingredient Tip:
For added texture, try using chunky peanut butter.

Nutrition (Per Serving):
Calories: 185 | Fat: 15g | Carbs: 8g | Net Carbs: 6g | Fiber: 2g | Protein: 7g

GARLIC AIOLI

This garlicky aioli feels fancy but is incredibly easy to make. Fresh herbs like chives and parsley add brightness, but they're optional.

30-Minute | One Pot | No Cook | Vegetarian
Serves: 4
Prep: 5 minutes + 30 minutes chilling

Ingredients:

- ½ cup mayonnaise

- 2 garlic cloves, minced

- Juice of 1 lemon

- 1 tablespoon chopped fresh flat-leaf Italian parsley

- 1 teaspoon chopped chives

- Pinch pink salt

- Freshly ground black pepper

Instructions:

1. In a food processor or blender, combine mayonnaise, garlic, lemon juice, parsley, and chives. Season with pink salt and pepper. Blend until fully combined.

2. Transfer to a sealed container and chill in the refrigerator for at least 30 minutes before serving. Store up to 1 week.

Ingredient Tip:
For best results, mince garlic very finely or grate it using a zester.

Nutrition (Per Serving):
Calories: 204 | Fat: 22g | Carbs: 3g | Net Carbs: 2g | Fiber: 1g | Protein: 1g

TZATZIKI

Tzatziki is a refreshing Mediterranean sauce, perfect as a dip or topping. The key is to remove excess water from the cucumber for the best texture.

No Cook | Vegetarian
Serves: 4
Prep: 10 minutes + at least 30 minutes chilling

Ingredients:

- ½ large English cucumber, unpeeled

- 1½ cups Greek yogurt (Fage recommended)

- 2 tablespoons olive oil

- Large pinch pink salt

- Large pinch freshly ground black pepper

- Juice of ½ lemon

- 2 garlic cloves, finely minced

- 1 tablespoon fresh dill

Instructions:

1. Cut the cucumber lengthwise and scoop out the seeds with a spoon.

2. Grate the cucumber using a zester or grater onto paper towels. Wrap the grated cucumber in the towels and squeeze out as much water as possible. (This step may take multiple paper towels or letting it drain overnight in a strainer or cheesecloth in the fridge.)

3. In a food processor or blender, combine the Greek yogurt, olive oil, pink salt, pepper, lemon juice, and garlic. Blend until smooth.

4. Transfer to a bowl and fold in the fresh dill and grated cucumber.

5. Chill for at least 30 minutes before serving. Store in a sealed container in the refrigerator for up to 1 week.

Ingredient Tip:
Mince garlic very finely for best flavor. Sour cream can be substituted for Greek yogurt if desired.

Nutrition (Per Serving):
Calories: 149 | Fat: 11g | Carbs: 5g | Net Carbs: 5g | Fiber: 1g | Protein: 8g

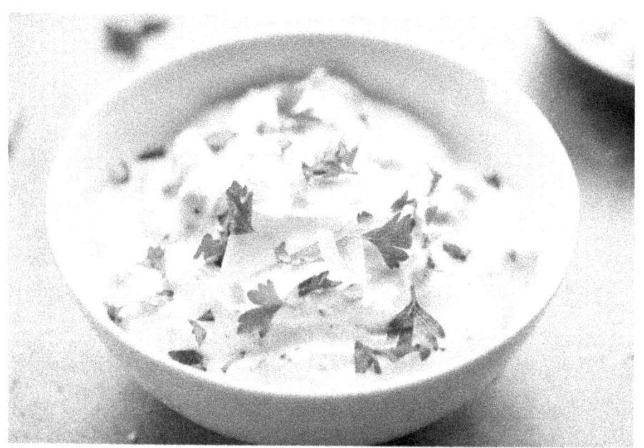

ALFREDO SAUCE

Rich, creamy Alfredo sauce is a comforting classic. Serve it over keto-friendly noodles like Miracle Noodles with grilled chicken and fresh herbs for a satisfying meal.

30-Minute | One Pot | Vegetarian
Serves: 2
Prep: 5 minutes
Cook: 10 minutes

Ingredients:

- 4 tablespoons butter

- 2 ounces cream cheese

- 1 cup heavy (whipping) cream

- ½ cup grated Parmesan cheese

- 1 garlic clove, finely minced

- 1 teaspoon dried Italian seasoning

- Pinch pink salt

- Freshly ground black pepper

Instructions:

1. In a medium saucepan over medium heat, combine butter, cream cheese, and heavy cream. Whisk constantly until the butter and cream cheese have melted and are fully incorporated.

2. Stir in Parmesan cheese, garlic, and Italian seasoning. Continue whisking until the sauce is smooth.

3. Reduce heat to medium-low and simmer gently for 5 to 8 minutes, stirring occasionally, until the sauce thickens.

4. Season with pink salt and pepper, stirring well to combine.

5. Toss with your favorite cooked keto-friendly noodles and serve immediately.

6. Store any leftovers in a sealed container in the refrigerator for up to 4 days.

Ingredient Tip:
Try using a blend of Parmesan, Asiago, and Romano cheeses for extra depth of flavor.

Nutrition (Per Serving):
Calories: 294 | Fat: 30g | Carbs: 2g | Net Carbs: 2g | Fiber: 0g | Protein: 5g

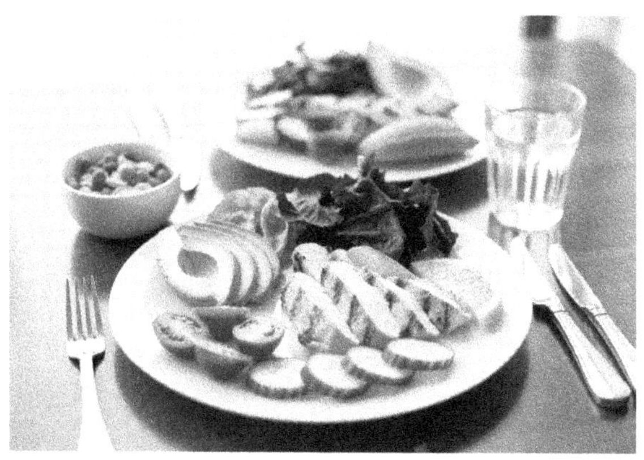

CONCLUSION

Embarking on a low-carb or ketogenic lifestyle can be both rewarding and empowering, especially when you have the right tools and knowledge at your fingertips. This book has aimed to provide you with practical, delicious recipes and essential guidance—from wholesome meals and satisfying snacks to flavorful sauces and dressings—designed to fit seamlessly into your daily routine.

By choosing to prepare your own food and dressings, you gain full control over the quality and nutritional content of what you consume, helping you stay true to your health goals. Remember, small changes can lead to lasting results. Whether you are just starting or deepening your keto journey, embracing mindful choices and fresh ingredients will support your well-being every step of the way.

Thank you for letting this guide be part of your path to a healthier, happier you. Here's to good food, great health, and a vibrant life ahead!

ABOUT THE AUTHOR

Dr. Ben Bigs, PhD is a wellness advocate and passionate home cook with a deep interest in the practical application of nutrition for everyday life. He believes that healthy eating should be simple, sustainable, and enjoyable—not complicated or restrictive.

With a strong focus on low-carb, high-fat cooking, Dr. Ben develops recipes that are approachable for busy individuals and families, emphasizing real ingredients, minimal prep time, and maximum flavor. His work is inspired by the belief that food should nourish the body while fitting seamlessly into real-life schedules.

Through his recipes, Dr. Ben encourages readers to build confidence in the kitchen, make informed food choices, and discover that healthy cooking can be both effortless and satisfying.

When he's not creating recipes, Dr. Ben enjoys exploring ingredient pairings, simplifying classic dishes, and helping others find balance through mindful eating.

REFERENCES

Centers for Disease Control and Prevention. 2016. "Dietary Intake for Adults Aged 20 and Over." *National Center for Health Statistics.* https://www.cdc.gov/nchs/fastats/diet.htm.

Wilson, Jacob, and Ryan Lowery. 2017. *The Ketogenic Bible: The Authoritative Guide to Ketosis.* Victory Belt Publishing.

U.S. Department of Agriculture, Agricultural Research Service. *Pesticide Data Program Annual Summary.* Accessed 2026. https://www.ams.usda.gov/datasets/pdp.

Harvard T.H. Chan School of Public Health. *The Nutrition Source – Fats and Cholesterol.* Accessed 2026. https://www.hsph.harvard.edu/nutritionsource/what-should-you-eat/fats-and-cholesterol/.

National Institutes of Health, Office of Dietary Supplements. *Dietary Supplements for Weight Management.* Accessed 2026. https://ods.od.nih.gov/factsheets/WeightManagement-Consumer/.

Mayo Clinic. *Ketogenic diet: Is the high-fat, low-carb diet right for you?* Accessed 2026. https://www.mayoclinic.org/healthy-lifestyle/nutrition-and-healthy-eating/expert-answers/ketogenic-diet/faq-20460703.

World Health Organization. *Pesticide Residues in Food: What you need to know.* Accessed 2026. https://www.who.int/news-room/fact-sheets/detail/pesticide-residues-in-food.

The Academy of Nutrition and Dietetics. *Understanding Carbohydrates*. Accessed 2026. https://www.eatright.org/health/wellness/healthy-aging/und erstanding-carbohydrates.

Food and Drug Administration. *Tips for Washing Fruits and Vegetables*. Accessed 2026. https://www.fda.gov/food/buy-store-serve-safe-food/tips-w ashing-fruits-and-vegetables.

Precision Nutrition. *The Beginner's Guide to the Ketogenic Diet*. Accessed 2026. https://www.precisionnutrition.com/ketogenic-diet.

RECOMMENDED RESOURCES FOR FURTHER READING

Ketogenic Nutrition & Low-Carb Living
- *The Ketogenic Bible* — Jacob Wilson & Ryan Lowery
  A comprehensive, science-backed guide to ketosis and metabolic health.

- *The Art and Science of Low Carbohydrate Living* — Stephen D. Phinney, MD, PhD & Jeff S. Volek, PhD, RD
  A foundational text explaining how low-carb diets work in the body.

- *The Complete Ketogenic Diet for Beginners* — Amy Ramos
  A practical, beginner-friendly introduction to keto eating.

Health, Metabolism & Weight Management
- Harvard T.H. Chan School of Public Health — Nutrition Source
  https://www.hsph.harvard.edu/nutritionsource/
  Evidence-based nutrition education and research.

- National Institutes of Health (NIH) — Nutrition Research
  https://www.niddk.nih.gov/
  Reliable information on metabolism, obesity, and dietary patterns.

Food Quality & Ingredient Awareness
- Environmental Working Group (EWG)
  https://www.ewg.org/

Guides on produce safety, pesticides, and clean eating.

- USDA FoodData Central
https://fdc.nal.usda.gov/
Nutritional breakdowns of foods and ingredients.

Recipe Inspiration & Keto Tools

- Diet Doctor
https://www.dietdoctor.com/
Low-carb and keto recipes, meal plans, and visual food guides.

- Ruled.me
https://www.ruled.me/
Keto calculators, guides, and practical tips.

- MyFitnessPal
Carb tracking and macro monitoring tool.

Cooking Skills & Kitchen Confidence

- *Salt, Fat, Acid, Heat* — Samin Nosrat
A timeless guide to understanding flavor balance in cooking.

- Serious Eats — Food Science & Technique
https://www.seriouseats.com/
Technique-focused cooking education useful even for keto adaptations.

Medical & Safety Note for Readers

Readers managing medical conditions, pregnancy, or medication use should consult a qualified healthcare professional before making significant dietary changes.